Walter Lübeck • Frank Arjava Petter • William Lee Rand

The Spirit of Reiki

The Complete Handbook of the Reiki System

From Tradition to the Present
Fundamental, Lines of Transmission, Original Writings, Mastery, Symbols, Treatments, Reiki as a Spiritual Path in Life, and Much More

Translations by Christine M. Grimm

LOTUS PRESS
SHANGRI-LA

The information and exercises introduced in this book have been carefully researched and passed on to the best of our knowledge and consciousness. Despite this fact, neither the authors nor the publisher assume any type of liability for presumed or actual damages of any kind that might result from the direct or indirect application or use of the statements in this book. The information in this book is intended for interested readers and educational purposes. Neither the authors nor the publisher want the readers to diagnose or treat an illness by themselves. We therefore recommend visiting a medical professional for diagnosis and treatment of any illness.

First English Edition 2001

The Shangri-La Series is published in cooperation
with Schneelöwe Verlagsberatung, Federal Republic of Germany

Walter Lübeck's chapters translated from German by Christine M. Grimm
Cover design by Kuhn Graphik, Digitales Design, Zürich
Photos and graphs: on pages 149-188 by Shouya P. T. Grigg,
on pages 211-214 by Daniel Muschalik, on pages 78-79 by Peter Ehrhardt,
on page 84 by Klaus-Peter Hüsch, on page 88 by Ute Rossow
Japanese Typography by Chetna Kobayashi

ISBN: 0-914955-67-5
Library of Congress Catalog Number: 00-134076

Printed in USA

Table of Contents

Introduction

—by Frank Arjava Petter—

"No man is an island" were the famous words by the sixteenth century poet John Donne. Four hundred years later, his truth is still as valid as it ever was. Our world keeps getting smaller every day. The Internet, environmental concerns, politics, and international trade bring the many cultures of this wonderful planet increasingly closer. The trend of the 21st Century is "let's do it together."

One human being, one village, one city, or even one country can no longer live entirely on its own. Competitiveness—the desire to be the first, the best, the foremost, and only one—has simply become outdated as a "value." This desire may have been useful in the past. The concept of evolution describes a process from dependence toward independence, ultimately resulting in interdependence. Dependence is not a completely negative state; it indicates the ability to love, to be open toward others, to accept and appreciate the other individual's merit, to see our own shortcomings, and to acknowledge that we are not alone. Dependence is the first step toward love.

However, if we do not have the desire to want to succeed on our own, to stand on our own feet and live our own life, growth is not likely to occur. This applies on the personal, cultural, and international level. An independent person, an independent community is an attractive display of great strength and sheer power—a force that cannot be denied. The Western world has been greatly influenced over the past few decades by the power of positive thinking and the theory that we create our own reality. However, independence is not the final destination.

The next step, interdependence, has the ultimate goal of communication between individuals and nations, and the above factors that affect the environment of our lovely planet. The perfect analogy for the state of interdependence is the principle of light. The same light shines within each of us. It lights the path for every being, whether sentient or insentient, whatever its path may be. We just have to look at nature to see its marvelous interplay of forces. Wherever we turn our eyes, the oneness of all things is an inevitable truth. Even in the Reiki system, power, love, and light form one unified whole. Only the unity of the energies makes life truly worth living.

The ultimate truth results from these three concepts, yet it exists far beyond them. This essence of the ultimate truth is that nothing can be done unless the divine wills it. The Indian sage Ramakrishna Paramhansa suggests that we give God the authority over our lives: Let God sign all the important documents, and everything else will simply fall into place. My personal life experience has shown me that this is what needs to occur before a human being can become a vehicle of the divine.

This book marks a shift in the consciousness of the worldwide Reiki community. Its three authors—Walter Lübeck, William Rand, and Frank Arjava Petter—would like to invite you, dear reader, on a journey to the heart. It is a journey toward oneness, a journey toward loving, growing, and living together as one unified community.

In this Aquarian Age, the individual ego will not be able to survive. It has done its duty, played its part, and served its purpose. It has dreamed its own dream, but now we are awakening. Once we wake up, the dream loses its significance and is soon forgotten.

When Hawayo Takata brought Reiki to Hawaii in 1937, she probably did not realize the impact it was going to have on the West. This book is dedicated to the great gift, the gift of Reiki that Hawayo Takata presented to the Western world. Reiki has become the most frequently applied individual healing technique throughout the world. There is an even greater potential for the future. Reiki has spread all over the globe within a period of twenty years, and it will spread into the hearts of many more of our fellow human beings in the new millennium.

Several reasons can explain why the Reiki power has been able to bring the world together. The most obvious of all is that it is so simple. In Dr. Usui's own words, "everyone can learn and practice Reiki." The second reason is that Reiki brings results. The results are the healing of the physical, mental, and emotional bodies with all their states of pleasure, pain, health, and disease. Reiki heals the present, as well as the past and the future. It heals the healthy and the sick, the wealthy and the poor, and the young and the old. It heals the Hindu, the Christian, the Buddhist, the Muslim, and the Jew—no matter where they live and what they do. Reiki has transcended these divisions and brought together all religions, races, and people who live and love across the vast expanses of this planet.

Yet not every aspect of Reiki is filled with harmony and bliss. It appears that we need a dose of conflict, a burst of friction between each other, for learning to occur. In recent years, we have had quite a bit of elbow action in the worldwide Reiki community. Attempts by specific groups to trademark the Reiki terms and use of the word Reiki are just one example of the friction. As all of us who work in the healing arts know, the symptom of a disease is not the disease itself. The symptom is just one small part of the disease, requiring us to uncover the cause and heal it in its many layers. With this book, we would like to offer the benefits of our healing work to all of you.

The three of us have totaly distinct views about Reiki, but we share the same vision of transcendence and the same experience of the Reiki energy. Our mutual vision of transcendence is the transcendence of opinions, the transcendence of our differences in favor of what is essential to all of us. We all share the experience of the life force that permeates everything—Reiki.

So we bring our vision to you, dear reader. You are also a part of the same energy. If the three of us can pool our energies and work toward one common goal, you can do the same with other individuals. This book beckons each of us to wake up from the dream of independence and personal action. Because the same energy makes all of our hearts beat, we might as well start working with each other instead of against each other. When two hands come together, the sense of individuality is transcended.

We are all one.

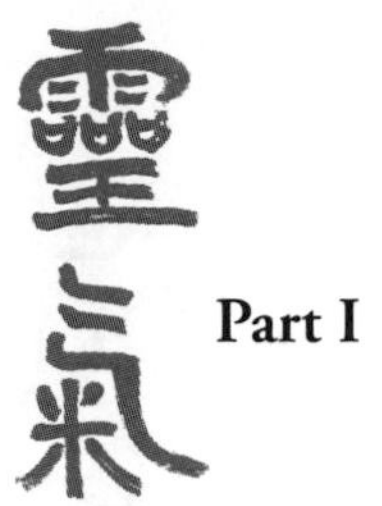

Part I

THE HISTORY OF REIKI

世の中に危きことはなかるべし
正しき道をふみたがへずば

: 115 ***The Road***

If you are walking
On the right path
No danger
Of this world
Will affect you

CHAPTER 1

Reiki in the Eastern World

—by William Lee Rand—

Reiki was discovered and developed by Dr. Mikao Usui, who was, among other things, a Japanese Buddhist monk. He was born in Japan on August 15, 1865 in the small village of Taniai in the Yamagata district of Gifu prefecture, located near present-day Nagoya.[1] Some have speculated that because he had traveled extensively and studied much, he may have come from a wealthy family. Although such is usually the case in Japan, it has not been confirmed.[1] My intuitive feeling is that his travels and studies were undertaken more in the style of a wandering monk who depended on personal initiative, flexibility, and divine providence than with the support of wealth.

We do know that at a young age, he studied *kiko* at a Tendai Buddhist temple on sacred Mt. Kurama, north of Kyoto. *Kiko* is the Japanese version of Qi Gong, a discipline designed to improve health through meditation, breathing practices, and slow moving exercises. It focuses on the development and use of *Ki* or life energy and includes methods for healing through the laying of hands.

Kiko requires that one build up a supply of healing energy through the use of the exercises before using it for healing. When using the kiko method, one is also prone to depletion, as it can draw on one's personal energy as well. The young Usui wondered if a way existed to heal without having to first store up healing energy and then leaving one depleted at the end. This was an important question and acted like a seed in his developing mind; a seed that would grow unnoticed until it suddenly came into fruition in a most profound way later in his life.[2]

Usui sensei traveled all over Japan, China, and Europe in pursuit of knowledge. He was intent on learning and studied a wide range of subjects, including medicine, psychology, religion, and spiritual development[1]. Because of his enhanced psychic abilities, he was able to join a metaphysical group called the *Rei Jyutu Ka*, where his education about the spiritual world continued.[3] His intense and continuing interest in knowledge created the foundation that allowed him to comprehend the significance of the amazing blessing that came to him years later.

His education and well-organized mind helped him get a job as the secretary of Shinpei Goto, then head of the department of health and welfare and later Mayor of Tokyo. One of the benefits of his job as secretary was getting to know many influential people all over Japan. The contacts helped him start his own business, and he eventually became a successful businessman.[4]

His business career went well for quite a while, but in 1914 it took a turn for the worse[3]. Having some knowledge of Buddhism, he decided to become a Buddhist monk. He focused his mind on the devotional practice and trained intensely. Eventually, he returned to Mt. Kurama where he had studied as a boy. He decided to take a twenty-one day retreat on the mountain.[1, 4] There he fasted, chanted, prayed, and meditated. One of the meditations he may have done involved standing under a small artificial waterfall and allowing the stream to fall on his head. This meditation is still practiced on Mt. Kurama to this day! Its purpose is to purify and open the crown chakra.

Toward the end of his retreat in March 1922, a great and powerful spiritual light entered the top of his head and he had a satori or enlightening experience. This light was the Reiki energy coming to him in the form of an attunement. His awareness was then greatly expanded, and he realized that a great power had entered him. He knew it was the power he had wished for when he had studied healing on Mt. Kurama as a child. He was overjoyed. He knew he could heal others without his energy being depleted.[1]

Usui sensei used Reiki on himself at first and then on members of his family. He moved to Tokyo in April 1922 and started a healing society that he named, "Usui Reiki Ryoho Gakkai" in English this means "Usui Reiki Healing Society." He also opened a clinic in Harajuku, Aoyama near the Meiji shrine in central Tokyo and began teaching classes and giving Reiki treatments.[1]

He then developed six levels or degrees for his training (according to Fumio Ogawa). He numbered his levels in reverse of what we do in the west: The first level was number six and the highest level was number one. (The first four levels, which were levels six to three, are what Mrs Takata taught as Reiki I. She combined all four into one degree. This is why she gave four attunements for her level one, one attunement for each level.) The first four levels were called *Shoden* or *beginning level*; the fifth level was called *Okuden* or *Inner teaching* and was divided into *Okuden Zenki* (first half) and *Okuden Koki* (second half); and the master level was called *Shinpiden*, or Mystery Teaching.[3]

Note that "master" was not used by Usui sensei and is not used in Japan. It was Hawayo Takata who created this title when she began teaching the Shinpiden level in 1970. It would have been wiser not to choose that term as in spiritual practices "master" denotes one who has become enlightened, a great spiritual accomplishment few on this planet have achieved. The *Shinpiden* level of Reiki is simply passed from the *Shinpiden* to the student without the student needing to be enlightened or even very spiritually developed when compared to an enlightened master. So, when people first began to hear about Reiki and about the Reiki master level, some thought it meant that a Reiki master is comparable to a spiritual master or enlightened master and so had a misconception about the spiritual condition of a Reiki master. In addition some wanted to become Reiki masters because of the status, rather than the value of passing Reiki on to others.

If the *Shinpiden* level had continued to be called *Shinpiden* in the west or had been simply called Reiki teacher, Reiki would not have had as much of the ego-grasping delusion that surrounded it when the master level first was taught in the West in the 70s and 80s.

Usui sensei continued teaching and giving treatments in the Tokyo clinic, but the peace and harmony was shaken in 1923 by the great Kanto earthquake, one of the worst and most devastating earthquakes to hit Japan. Over 140,000 people were killed. Thousands of houses and buildings crumbled to the ground, and many more burned in the ensuing fire. Thousands of people were left homeless, and many others were injured or became physically ill. Almost everyone was emotionally traumatized.[5] The demand for Reiki became enormous and Usui sensei and his students worked night and day to help as many as they could. In 1925, he opened a much larger clinic in Nakano, Tokyo and began traveling all over Japan to spread the word about Reiki. The need for healing after the earthquake continued for many years, and during that span Usui sensei taught Reiki to over two thousand students and trained sixteen teachers.[1] "Because of the help he provided, the Japanese government recognized him with the Kun San To award for meritorious service to others." [4]

Usui sensei did not want Reiki to be the exclusive practice of just one group or to be controlled or limited in any way. Rather, he wanted it to be available to everyone and to spread throughout the world. He thought Reiki was a way for anyone to experience the divine, and because of this, people would then be more willing to work together to create a better world.[6, 8]

Usui sensei passed over on March 9, 1926 after suffering a stroke while teaching a Reiki class in Fukuyama. He is buried at the Saihoji Temple in Suginami-Ku, Tokyo. After his death, his students erected a large memorial stone next to his grave with a beautiful inscription describing his life and his work with Reiki.

When Usui sensei discovered Reiki, many other hands-on healing methods were being taught. According to Toshitaka Mochizuki, the Taireidou healing technique was started by Morihei Tanaka and *Tenohira-Ryouchi-Kenkyukai*, which means "The Association for The Study of Palm Treatments," was started by Toshihiro Eguchi, who learned healing from Usui Sensei before founding his own group. Eguchi also wrote books on healing, which are now difficult to find. Jintai-Ragium-Gakkai, which means "The Human Body Radium Society," was founded by Chiwake Matsumoto. *Shinnoukyou-Honin* was a religious group founded by Taikan Nishimura, whose method was called Shinnoukyou-Syokushu-Shikou Ryoho, meaning "Violet Light Healing Method." Also the religions Mahi Kari and Johrei started in Japan, and both have a central focus of healing with the hands. Interestingly, both use the same symbol that Usui sensei chose for the master symbol. I do not know if any connection exists between these healing systems, but their nearly simultaneous beginnings indicate a sudden increase in interest toward healing all over Japan at the time Usui sensei discovered Reiki.

After Usui sensei passed, Mr. J. Ushida became president of the Usui Reiki Ryoho Gakkai and he took the initiative to erect the Usui memorial and wrote the inscription. Below is a list of the presidents of the Usui Reiki Ryoho Gakkai and the approximate dates that they served.*

Presidents of the Usui Reiki Ryoho Gakkai	
Dr. Mikao Usui	1922 – 1926
Mr. Juzaburo Ushida	1926 – 1935
Mr. Kan'ichi Taketomi	1935 – 1960
Mr. Yoshiharu Watanabe	? – 1960
Mr. Hoichi Wanami	? – 1975
Mrs. Kimiko Koyama	1975 – 1999
Mr. Masayoshi Kondo	1999 – today

Here is a list of seven of the sixteen teachers that Usui sensei trained. The list comes from the research of Frank Arjava Petter and Dave King:

Toshihiro Eguchi
Ilichi Taketomi
Toyoichi Wanami
Yoshiharu Watanabe
Kozo Ogawa
Juzaburo Ushida
Chujiro Hayashi

You may be surprised to see that while Dr. Chujiro Hayashi received his *Shinpiden* degree from Dr. Usui, he was never president of the *Usui Reiki Ryoho Gakkai*. After Usui sensei passed, Dr. Hayashi broke away from the Gakkai to form his own association. He kept detailed records of all his treatments and developed his own style of Reiki that included special hand positions for treating various illnesses. His teaching manual, which includes the hand positions, can be found in chapter 19. While Dr. Hayashi was a respected Reiki master, and was president of his own organization, he was never the Grandmaster of the Usui system. In fact the title was never a part of Usui Reiki.

---

* These dates are derived from the understanding that the presidents served until they died.

CHAPTER 2

Reiki in the Western World

—by William Lee Rand—

Hawayo Takata was responsible for bringing Reiki to the west. Otherwise, Reiki would likely have taken a much longer time to leave Japan, if it would have left at all. Because of her, Reiki has spread all over the world and many millions of people have benefited from its healing power.

Hawayo Takata was born on December 24th, 1900 on the island of Kauai, Hawaii, and as she grew up, she began working at the sugar-cane plantations. She eventually married the accountant on one of the plantations, and after she gave birth to two children, her husband died in 1930. Hawayo Takata had to raise her children by herself, working in the sugar-cane fields to provide for her family. The work was very hard, and after five years she developed a lung condition and abdominal pains and had a nervous breakdown. One of her sisters died soon thereafter, and she traveled to Japan to visit her parents and seek help for her health.

She first went to a regular medical hospital, but then decided to try a different approach. She eventually went to Dr. Hayashi's Reiki clinic. She received two treatments a day, and after four months she was completely healed. Tests at a regular hospital confirmed it. She was very happy to be healed and wanted to learn Reiki to maintain her health when back in Hawaii. In 1936 she learned Shoden from Dr. Hayashi. She worked in his clinic doing Reiki treatments for a year and then received Okuden.

In 1937 she returned to Hawaii. Dr. Hayashi followed her and together they traveled around Hawaii giving lectures, teaching Reiki, and giving treatments. On February 21, 1938 Hawayo Takata was initiated into Shinpiden by Dr. Hayashi.[7]

Hawayo Takata established a clinic near Hilo, Hawaii and also had another one in Honolulu. She gave treatments and also trained students to Okuden, which she began calling Level II. She became a well-known healer and traveled to the U.S. mainland and to other parts of the world, teaching and giving treatments.

In 1970, she began training others in the Shinpiden, or master level as she began to call it. She charged $10,000 for the training, which was a weekend class without any apprenticeship*.

Hawayo Takata initiated twenty-two Reiki masters before her death on December 11, 1980**. She made all of them take a sacred oath to teach exactly as she had so as to preserve the Usui system, as she interpreted it. While the lineage went back to Dr. Usui, her teaching and practice method left out much of what Dr. Usui himself considered to be important and added many of her own rules. Some of these rules were felt to be restrictive and what she taught would, for sake of clarity, more appropriately be called "Takata Reiki."

The high fee she charged for the master level may have had some benefit, as it instilled a greater feeling of respect for Reiki. But not everyone felt this way. Some felt this to be an artificial way to create respect and by using money in such a way, it diverted attention away from the respect Reiki deserves because of the healing and other benefits it provides. The high fee also prevented many from receiving Reiki and prevented it from spreading very quickly. This went against the spirit of what Dr. Usui had wanted as it was his intention that Reiki be available to everyone and not be restricted to one select group, but that it spread around the world.[1, 6, 8]

After Hawayo Takata died, one of the twenty-two masters she had trained decided to disregard what she had required and to follow her own inner guidance. Iris Ishikura began charging a very moderate fee for the master level; in some cases she taught it free. Therefore, in the mid-80s, Reiki began to spread more quickly. By the end

---

* *Journey into Consciousness*, by Bethal Phaigh, page 130. That Hawayo Takata gave Reiki Master training in a weekend has been confirmed by other Masters she initiated.

** Hawayo Takata gave a list of the twenty-two Masters she initiated to her sister before she died. They are: George Araki, Dorothy Baba (deceased), Ursula Baylow, Rick Bockner, Barbara Brown, Fran Brown, Patricia Ewing, Phyllis Lei Furumoto, Beth Gray, John Gray, Iris Ishikura (deceased), Harry Kuboi, Ethel Lombardi, Barbara McCullough, Mary McFadyen, Paul Mitchell, Bethel Phaigh (deceased), Barbara Weber Ray, Shinobu Saito (Takata's sister), Virginia Samdahl, and Wanja Twan.

of the 80s probably several hundred Reiki masters charged modest fees. The number increased quickly, and now modest fees for the master level are the rule. Only a very small number of Reiki masters still charge $10,000.

I believe that Reiki students are guided to the teacher right for them. Because of this, the fee the teacher is charging is exactly the right fee for the student to pay. Those that paid $10,000 for the master level were supposed to pay it. Those who paid a lesser amount were supposed to pay the lesser amount also. Every teacher has the right to charge any amount or teach for free. The fee one pays for Reiki training does not affect the quality of the training. As we have seen, Hawayo Takata charged a very high amount for training in one weekend. For perspective, some Reiki teachers take a much longer time to train masters and charge less than Hawayo Takata did.

When Hawayo Takata introduced Reiki to the West, she added some rules that many consider restrictive and were not part of what Dr. Usui had taught. This may have made it more difficult for students to learn Reiki and also slowed its growth. This is explained in greater detail in the next chapter. However, it is important for us not to lose sight of the great value she created by bringing Reiki to the West. We are grateful for her contribution and continue to respect her for the wonderful blessings her work has brought to us. After Hawayo Takata passed, some teachers who loved Reiki began to modify the restrictions she had added and began to follow their inner guidance and to teach more openly—including allowing their students to take notes and tape record.

They also began supplying written material and class workbooks and charging more moderate fees. Others began to research the history of Reiki. Eventually, new information from Japan about Dr. Usui's life and how he taught began to show up. The new information that came from documented evidence confirmed what most had felt all along—that Reiki should be taught openly and made available to everyone. We are thankful that those with the courage to follow their inner guidance have done so. Because of this, his dream of Reiki becoming available to all people of the world is quickly becoming a reality.

The Evolution of Reiki

One of the qualities of the Western mind is to seek to make improvements. Progress seems to be a cultural necessity, and we are always trying to make things bigger, more powerful, or enhanced in some way. This process has not stopped with Reiki. Once Reiki reached the West and especially since it became more easily available in the 80s and 90s, Reiki students have had a field day with the new technique.

Out of inspiration and from a desire to provide greater benefit, people were guided toward new methods to meet modern needs. Many have channeled new symbols and developed variations for the attunement process. Many sensitive people realized that the new healing techniques that had been channeled still had the same core qualities of Usui Reiki Ryoho; the vibration of the healing energy was just different. While it is true that all healing comes from one source, it became apparent that Reiki can come in different "flavors," with different effects.

Some of the qualities people have noticed in the newer variations of Reiki are being more grounded and coming from the earth or having a lighter quality and coming from the universe, or being softer, gentler, more powerful, denser, more refined, etc. It was also noticed that the new Reiki energy seemed to work better than Usui Reiki Ryoho for some healing situations. Some of the new Reiki systems also include new symbols that bring in healing energies with a specific purpose or benefit. These include the ability to relieve pain, heal deeply, create grounding, open the heart, create peace, inspire, enhance creativity, manifest goals, protect, etc.

Having several kinds of Reiki to work with and additional symbols gives the practitioner greater flexibility and allows healing to take place more quickly and often with better results. The situation is similar to a repair person fixing up a home. If all the person has is a screw driver, a hammer, and a pair of pliers, he or she can make some improvements. But if the person adds a saw, a set of wood chisels, wire cutters, and a set of wrenches, he or she can quickly accomplish much more. Many have found an advantage to having several different kinds of Reiki to work with.

When differences in the qualities of the new healing energies were noticed, people realized a different kind of Reiki was being channeled and gave the practice a new name. The first of the new Reiki techniques was called Mari el®, channeled in 1983 by Ethel Lombardi, who was one of Hawayo Takata's masters. Many others followed, including The Radiance Technique®, Raku Kei, Tibetan Reiki, Karuna Reiki®, Rainbow Reiki, Golden Age Reiki, Reiki Jin-Kei Do®, Satya Japanese Reiki, Men Chho Reiki®, Jinlap Reiki, Seichim, Saku Reiki, Blue Star Reiki, Reiki Plus®—and the list continues. There are now over 30 different kinds of Reiki with many subgroups and branches, and more are being channeled all the time.

A Definition of Reiki

Some people become confused when they hear of different kinds of Reiki, as they believe that Reiki is what Dr. Usui channeled—any other healing technique should have another name. When Dr. Usui was given the new healing technique, the word Reiki was already in use in Japan. Dr. Usui did not call his technique *Reiki*. He called it *Usui Reiki Ryoho* to make sure people understood it was a unique kind of Reiki. With the channeling of other healing methods similar to *Usui Reiki Ryoho*, but with different vibrations and effects, it has become clear that there is now a whole class of healing methods that can appropriately be called Reiki.

With this in mind, how can one tell what is a Reiki technique and what is not? By analyzing the Reiki given to Dr. Usui, we find four unique qualities that identify the class of healing techniques appropriately called Reiki. These four qualities may be defined in the following way:

1. The ability to perform Reiki comes from receiving an attunement, rather than developing the ability over time through the use of meditation or other exercises.
2. All Reiki techniques are part of a lineage, meaning the technique has been passed from teacher to student through an attunement process, starting with the one who first channeled the technique.

3. Reiki does not require that one guides the energy with the mind, as it is guided by the higher power that knows what vibration or combination of vibrations to have and how to act.
4. Reiki can do no harm.

If a healing technique has these four qualities, it can be considered to be a Reiki technique.

CHAPTER 3

Hawayo Takata's Reiki Story

—by William Lee Rand—

When I first began to research the history of Reiki and realized that there were serious problems with the story Hawayo Takata had told, I became disillusioned. At that time, no one in the West knew where Dr. Usui's grave was located, and we had no Reiki contacts in Japan. Hawayo Takata had supplied the only information available. When her story began to unravel, I began to wonder if Dr. Usui had ever existed and thought that perhaps the whole story had been made up. Because of this, I wondered if I should continue to practice Reiki; I was in a spiritual dilemma. But after meditating on the situation, I realized experience indicated Reiki to be a valid healing method and because of this I should continue practicing it, and at the same time continue my research in hopes that more of the story would unfold and the real Dr. Usui would be discovered. I also wondered why Hawayo Takata decided to change the story of Reiki. In speculating about this, I realized that World War II started just after Hawayo Takata brought Reiki to the West. In fact the war started when the Japanese attacked Pearl Harbor in Hawaii where Hawayo Takata lived and was teaching Reiki. The opinion about anything Japanese suddenly became very low. People did not trust anything that came from Japan and made fun of everything Japanese. Also, many people of Japanese descent were placed in internment camps. The conditions in these camps were very poor; there was no freedom and the people were treated like prisoners. Fortunately, Hawayo Takata was able to avoid the internment camp. But even so, this must have been a very challenging time for her and it must have been very difficult to promote a Japanese practice like Reiki. So, perhaps she decided that the only way she could continue practicing Reiki was to make the founder of Reiki appear to be more of a Westerner. Perhaps this is why she said that Dr. Usui had been a Christian minister and that he had attended a University in the United States and that he had been president of a Christian University in Japan. This could also be the reason she made so many other changes to the way she practiced.

The following information is stated in a very direct way and some may feel that it casts a derogatory light on Hawayo Takata's integrity. However, I believe she did the best she could during very trying circumstances. It is important for us to focus on the positive things she did and to respect and honor her for bringing Reiki to the West and for continuing to practice and teach it during such a difficult time.

To date, over sixty books have been written about Reiki. The history of Reiki that has appeared in most of them is the story of Reiki Hawayo Takata told. The story, available on an audio-tape recording and transcript made prior to her transition, has usually been repeated verbatim by most authors. Many people wonder why so many authors continue to do so when the facts do not support her story. Part of the reason is that many of these books were written before the facts became well known.

Nevertheless, it is unusual that an author would repeat a story without taking the time to research it, but apparently that is what happened with writings on Reiki. When writing about history, it is important not to simply accept a story someone has told, but to research it to verify the facts wherever possible. Historical research is usually based on original documents and multiple interviews with people, or organizations who have firsthand experience, in order to develop an understanding that is supported from several different directions.

As an example, Hawayo Takata stated that Dr. Usui had been the president of Doshisha University in Kyoto, Japan. It would be a relatively simple matter for any author to contact Doshisha University to verify this piece of information before stating it as fact. Unfortunately, most previous authors have not done this. A few recent authors have undertaken this extra step. As her story was researched by Arjava Petter, Chetna Kobayashi, myself, and others, it became increasingly evident that the Takata story of Reiki had many weaknesses and "mythological" elements not based on historical fact. Because the Takata history of Reiki has been included in so many Reiki books, I will not repeat it entirely here. However, for the benefit of all those familiar with her story, I think it is important to go over her story and supply the facts as we now know them to be, based on authentic research. You will then have a more accurate version of the history and will understand the way the Takata story has influenced the practice of Reiki in the West.

Hawayo Takata said, in flyers she used to advertise her classes, that she was the only Reiki master in the world. She also stated that all Reiki masters in Japan had died in the war. This was also part of the story told by many of her students and by the two Reiki organizations started by her students after she died. This part of her story is important because anyone wanting to research Reiki beyond the Takata story, would have been discouraged from doing so as it leaves Hawayo Takata, and her story appearing to be the only source of information about the history of Reiki.

While many who heard this part of her story were doubtful, because of geographic, cultural, and language barriers, it was difficult for those in the West to research the history of Reiki. Most accepted it because it was the only information available.

It is now known that Reiki masters always existed and practiced in Japan both during and after the war. In fact Reiki has been continuously practiced in Japan and represented by the Reiki organization started by Dr. Usui, the *Usui Reiki Ryoho Gakkai*, located in Tokyo. Based on our research, the president of the organization during the war was Mr. Kanichi Taketomi, and he remained president until his death in 1960.

It is also known that Hawayo Takata had contact with at least several of the masters in Japan after the war. As an example, Dr. Hayashi's wife, Chie Hayashi, who was a Reiki master and a friend of Hawayo Takata, continued to practice and teach Reiki in Japan after the war. I have corresponded with a woman in Hawaii, Yoshi Kimura, whose father Tatseyi Nagao had received first- and second-degree Reiki from Hawayo Takata in Hawaii. In 1950, her father went to Japan to receive the *Shinpiden* level from Chie Hayashi. He returned to Hawaii to practice and teach Reiki until he died at age 96 in 1980, the same year Hawayo Takata passed. So it is clear that

Hawayo Takata had contact with other Reiki masters after the war, even one who had taken classes from her and lived close to her clinic in Hawaii.

Hawayo Takata stated that Reiki is an oral tradition and therefore no written material should be given to Reiki students. She did not allow taking notes and tape recording. The rule was strictly enforced and passed on as a necessary part of the Usui system of Reiki to all the masters she trained.

We now know that this idea was not universally accepted. Reiki is not solely an oral tradition. Both Dr. Usui and Dr. Hayashi had written material they gave to their students. We have copies of both their teaching manuals, which contain many important exercises and also include hand positions for treating specific illnesses. Frank Arjava Petter has published a translation of Dr. Usui's manual in his books.[6, 8] and a translation of Dr. Hayashi's handbook is included at the back of this book (s. chapter 19, pages 190 ff).

We know that Hawayo Takata had Dr. Hayashi's manual, as she gave copies of it to some of her students. Not having written material and not being able to take notes or tape record made it more difficult for students to learn. Beginning in the late 1980s, several teachers used their own common sense and allowed their students to take notes and tape record and provided handouts and instruction manuals. This is now a common practice.

Hawayo Takata said she was the representative of Usui Reiki and she taught an unaltered form of Usui Reiki, the same as taught by Dr. Usui. From a handbook written by Mrs. Kimiko Koyama we know about many exercises Dr. Usui taught, but Hawayo Takata didn't. Hawayo Takata knew about at least some of these exercises, as she mentions them in her diary. In her diary entry dated May 1936, she states: "What was more than pleasing was that Mr. Hayashi has granted to bestow upon me the secret of Shinpiden, Kokyu-Ho and the Reiji-Ho, the ultimate in the energy science."

According to Hawayo Takata, she learned Reiki in Japan from Dr. Hayashi in 1935. We have discovered that Dr. Hayashi broke away from the *Usui Reiki Ryoho Gakkai* and created his own form of Reiki, making important changes from what he had learned from Dr. Usui and what was being taught by the Gakkai. The changes may have been beneficial, but by making them, he created his own style of Reiki. Further, he called his Reiki clinic the Hayashi Reiki Institute. The idea that Hawayo Takata taught Usui Reiki is the basis for her followers calling themselves "traditional" Usui Reiki practitioners and for stating that they have an authentic form of Usui Reiki.

Hawayo Takata also stated that she was the successor to Dr. Hayashi and was in charge of his clinic etc. According to information from Mrs. Yamagouchi in Kyoto, Japan, it was Chie Hayashi who became Dr. Hayashi's successor. Mrs. Yamagouchi was a Reiki master initiated by Dr. Hayashi in 1938 who, as of this writing continues to practice and teach Reiki in Japan.

Hawayo Takata did not practice "traditional" Usui Reiki, but a variation developed by Dr. Hayashi in which she left out many exercises she knew were apart of the Usui system. It is also believed that Hawayo Takata further modified the style of Reiki she practiced after Dr. Hayashi died. I consider it unfortunate that she chose, for whatever reasons, not to teach the Usui system of Reiki, as now that we have had a chance to practice the exercises from Dr. Usui's handbook, we are finding that they are very helpful.

Hawayo Takata stated that Dr. Usui was a Christian. Quoting from the transcript of her recorded history she says, "At this time in the beginning of the story Dr. Usui was the principal of the Doshisha University in Kyoto. Also minister on Sunday, and at the University they had a chapel. So he was a full-fledged Christian minister . . ." According to the Gakkai, Dr. Usui had never been a Christian; he was a Buddhist. Dr. Usui is buried at Saihoji temple, a (Pure Land) Buddhist temple. If he had been a Christian, he would have been buried at a Christian cemetery. Doshisha University has no record of Dr. Usui having been the president, a faculty member, or a student; in fact, the school has no knowledge of him at all. (See the letter from Doshisha University in the back of this book on page 303.)

Hawayo Takata said that Dr. Usui had enrolled in the University of Chicago in the United States and completed his studies to receive a degree in theology. But when checking with the University of Chicago, we found they could not locate any information to verify that he had taken even one class from the school or the Lutheran college from which the University of Chicago was established. (See the letter from the University of Chicago in the back of this book on page 304.)

Did Dr. Usui Have Another Name?

One of the reasons some say that we can't find a record of Dr. Usui being the president of Doshisha University or attending the University of Chicago is that he used another name. This speculation is however unlikely and we could find no evidence to support this idea. Usui is the name on his gravestone at Saihoji cemetery. It is also his family name as verified by the names of family members buried there and by living members of his family. (While his memorial stone states that he had a second name of Gyoho, this is a name for use in the afterlife and was not used by him during his lifetime.) I It would be highly unlikely for a Japanese person to use a name other than his family name if he were president of a University or had registered at a University as a student.

Hawayo Takata said Dr. Usui rediscovered Reiki in a formula in one of the Buddhist sutras that he read in Sanskrit at a Zen temple. She did not state which sutra this was, and no one has been able to find a formula for acquiring Reiki in any of the Buddhist sutras. We have been unable to therefore verify this statement, and, while possible, it appears not to be entirely consistent with statements made by Dr. Usui himself.

Dr. Usui said that Reiki is an original form of healing. In his handbook, the *Reiki Ryoho Hikkei*, Dr. Usui states "Our Reiki Ryoho is something absolutely original and cannot be compared with any other [spiritual] path in the world." Later he said, "First of all, our Reiki Ryoho is an original therapy, which is built upon the spiritual power of the universe." Inscribed on the Usui memorial stone it says that the system of Reiki came from Dr. Usui's mystical experience on Mt. Kurama.

The only source of information that says that Dr. Usui rediscovered Reiki is from Hawayo Takata, and we have already seen that other parts of her Reiki history are not entirely factual. I personally think that Dr. Usui's own words are a more accurate source of information about where Reiki came from. From this we can conclude that Dr. Usui did not rediscover Reiki, but that it is an original form of healing that he developed. Of course the energy of Reiki, may have been part of one or more healing systems previously practiced. However, it appears that Dr. Usui had a powerful mystical experience on Mt. Kurama in which he received Reiki healing energy directly from the source. From the experience he developed the Reiki healing system.

Hawayo Takata also stated that the official fee for Reiki mastership was $10,000; if one did not charge the amount, one was not practicing the Usui system of Reiki. In the Reiki organization started by some of Hawayo Takata's students, the need to pay $10,000 for your Reiki mastership is emphasized; often as the most important point. The fee was one of the greatest restrictions to the spread of Reiki, especially in the early 80s, as most of those teaching Reiki in the West were charging it. Now that we have additional information from Japan, it is apparent that the $10,000 fee for Reiki mastership was not a part of the Usui system per se, but rather the fee established by Hawayo Takata herself. According to Mr. Doi, the Japanese Gakkai, of which he is a member, charges very moderate fees. They have a lifetime-membership fee of $100 and a $20 fee for each meeting one attends. Also, according to Mrs. Yamagouchi, the fee she paid for her mastership from Dr. Hayashi was equal to about one months pay. This was not a small amount, but certainly not the $10,000 required by Hawayo Takata.

Following in Takata's Footsteps

After Hawayo Takata died in December 1980, Barbara Weber Ray claimed to be the Grandmaster of Reiki. She said that Hawayo Takata had wanted her to take charge of Reiki after she passed and that she was the Grandmaster. Then another woman, Phyillis Furumoto, made the same claim. Two separate Reiki organizations were started around them, and both claimed that their leaders were the Grandmaster of Reiki, which they both continue to claim to this day! (Phyllis Furumoto may be the successor to Hawayo Takata's legacy, as she claims, but as previously explained Hawayo Takata was never in charge of the Usui system, nor was she the successor to Dr. Hayashi.)

It is important to note that neither Hawayo Takata, Dr. Hayashi, nor Dr. Usui called themselves Grandmaster. The title only came into use in the West after Hawayo Takata died. It has never been used in Japan. Reportedly, Dr. Usui was a very humble man. He himself, said, was not on the highest energy level. He graded himself as number Two, leaving the possibility for further development widely open.

As previously stated, the organization started by Dr. Usui is called the *Usui Reiki Ryoho Gakkai* and it is headquartered in Tokyo, Japan. Dr. Usui was the first president of the Usui Reiki Ryoho Gakkai, and when he died, Mr. Juzaburo Ushida became president. It was Mr. Ushida who was responsible for erecting the Usui Memorial stone next to Dr. Usui's grave at Saihoji Temple. Dr. Hayashi was never the president and in fact could not have become president because he broke away from the Usui organization to start his own group. Therefore, no one in Dr. Hayashi's lineage could have become the president of the Usui organization. At the time that Barbara Weber Ray and Phyllis Furumoto were claiming to be the Grandmaster of Reiki, Mrs. Kimiko Koyama was president of the *Usui Reiki Ryoho Gakkai.* The person currently in charge of the *Usui Reiki Ryoho Gakkai* is Mr. Masayoshi Kondo, who lives in Tokyo, Japan.

So, as you can see, based on factual evidence, Hawayo Takata did not teach the same style of Reiki that Dr. Usui taught, and she was not part of the organization Dr. Usui started. She could not have been in charge of the Usui system of Reiki and neither can any of her students. However, her contributions to the introduction and teaching of Reiki in the West are nevertheless extremely valuable in their own right, and she certainly introduced Reiki to a great many people.

For some, this imformation may come as a shock as there has been so much emphasis placed on Hawayo Takata being in charge of the Usui system and teaching Usui Reiki in an unaltered way. I know it effected me this way when I first began hear about it. However, these events have had no effect on the quality of Reiki energy and now that we have a factual basis for the history of Usui Reiki and its original methods, it can be presented in a more professional way. Furthermore, the factual story makes it much easier for all Reiki groups to work together in harmony.

Reiki has survived and spread all over the planet even with the obvious limitations mentioned above. It is a tribute to the remarkable power of Reiki and indicates that this healing energy is authentic and able to overcome the challanges and momentary concerns of past teachers. We are grateful to all those who have contributed to its preservation and to uncovering its original methods and intent. May the spirit of Reiki continue to grow so that the healing, happiness and peace it offers can be experienced by everyone in our beautiful world.

CHAPTER 4

What is Reiki Tradition?

—by Frank Arjava Petter—

The *American Heritage Dictionary of the English Language* defines tradition as:

1 The passing down of elements of a culture from generation to generation, especially by oral communication.
2 a) A mode of thought or behavior followed by a people continuously from generation to generation; a custom or usage.
2 b) A set of such customs and usages viewed as a coherent body of precedents influencing the present: followed family tradition in dress and manners.
3 A body of unwritten religious precepts.
4 A time-honored practice or set of such practices.
5 Law: Transfer of property to another.

The root of the word tradition has its origins in the Latin word "traditus, (the) past participle of (the verb) *tradere*, to hand over, deliver, entrust."

People often speak of the "Reiki tradition," "Traditional Reiki," "in the tradition of Dr. Usui," and so forth. But, as a matter of fact, none of us in the West know much about the true Reiki tradition! Our twenty years or so of Western Reiki tradition have been based upon Hawayo Takata's understanding of it. Many people, not just one individual, usually carry on a tradition. As a result, research into the background of a tradition can be done easily and successfully. In the case of Western Reiki, it is hard to determine exactly what happened between Dr. Usui and Dr. Hayashi and between Dr. Hayashi and Hawayo Takata because all of the people involved have now passed away. Research in Japan suggests that Dr. Hayashi was considered a "bad boy" among the *Usui Reiki Ryoho Gakkai*. After all, he broke away from the main group and started his own system. We can be glad he did; otherwise, none of us in the West would have had the chance to learn Reiki!

After the Eastern and Western Reiki paths parted—from the early 1940s to the mid-1980s—the strangest thing happened: Western students of Reiki were told that there were no living Reiki practitioners in Japan. They were told that Hawayo Takata had been the only practicing Reiki Master in the world. They were also informed that all the Japanese Reiki practitioners had died in World War II! Though it may sound absurd, I know it could have been possible because I was born in Dusseldorf, a German city that was basically wiped off the face of the earth during World War II. The Reiki practitioners could have all died in Hiroshima or Nagasaki. But the fact was that Japanese Reiki has survived until the present day.

As more and more original Reiki manuscripts are discovered in Japan, we may be forced to reconsider what we call Reiki tradition. One possible step would be to use the name of "Hayashi-Takata Reiki" instead of Usui Reiki for Western Reiki. A Japanese Reiki teacher with whom I spoke several years ago proposed the term after he heard that Phyllis Furumoto had tried to copyright the word Reiki. Fortunately, the absurd venture has since been scrapped.

A more positive approach would be to incorporate the "new" aspects of the original Japanese Reiki into Western Reiki as we advance on our path of discovery. Many facts and facets of Dr. Usui's life and work have recently come to light. His original Reiki techniques have been discovered and are now being used by thousands of Reiki practitioners worldwide. However, the one vital aspect of Reiki work that still remains a mystery to us is the initiation or attunement process employed by Dr. Usui.

As of today, I am not aware of anyone in the Western world who knows exactly how Dr. Usui and the modern Usui Reiki Ryoho Gakkai attunes and initiates members into Reiki.

Many Reiki teachers in Japan in the meantime offer to teach what they call the original Usui Reiki Ryoho Gakkai *Rei Ju* (attunement) technique for. However, I know for a fact that what is being taught is Mr. Doi's version of *Rei Ju.* Although Mr. Doi makes it very clear in his workshops that what he teaches is his own technique, some of his students prefer to overlook that statement. In 1999 I attended one of his workshops in Vancouver; afterwards, several participants started offering their students the "original Gakkai attunement process." When will we ever learn?

Until one of the Usui Reiki Ryoho Gakkai Reiki Masters (of which there are only six)—or some member of another group in Japan—comes forth and shares the knowledge with us, we are simply dealing with guesswork. Guesswork is not satisfying in the least.

William, Walter, and I are committed to continue searching and researching in Japan. Maybe you are also interested. We are certain that someone will succeed one day, and we look forward to the celebration ...

CHAPTER 5

Contemporary Reiki in Japan

—by Frank Arjava Petter—

After Dr. Usui's death, the Japanese Reiki movement split into several groups, including Dr. Hayashi's *Hayashi Shiki Reiki Ryoho*. We do know that Dr. Hayashi broke away from the *Usui Reiki Ryoho Gakkai* at some point because he called his own system *Hayashi Shiki Reiki Ryoho* (see chapter 19 on the *Hayashi Shiki Handbook* on pages 188 ff) and not Usui Reiki. Another fact leads us to the same conclusion: We were all taught that Mr. Hayashi gave the Reiki Master/Teacher degree to Hawayo Takata. However, the Usui Reiki Ryoho Gakkai does not permit anyone except their president to bestow the title, even though teachers like Mr. Hayashi were allowed to have their own students.

Little is known about the facts of why and when Dr. Hayashi departed from the circle of the Usui Reiki Ryoho Gakkai. It may have been after Dr. Usui died. In many traditions circumstances often change when the originator of the system dies.

It is said that Dr. Hayashi became quite famous in his day and the size of his group actually greatly exceeded the original Usui Reiki Ryoho Gakkai. Mr. Doi, a member of the Gakkai, told me that the Hayashi Shiki Reiki Ryoho disappeared with the death of Chujiro Hayashi, who committed suicide in 1941. However, American sources tell that Ms. Hayashi kept teaching Reiki after her husband's death.

According to sources in Japan, the mystical story of Dr. Hayashi's "internal suicide" that many of us have read in Western Reiki books is a fairy tale. Following Dr. Hayashi's affiliation with Hawayo Takata in the 1930s, Hawayo Takata frequently traveled to the United States. World War II broke out in the meantime, and America became Japan's enemy. Rumors in Japan say he chose to terminate his own life because he was suspected of being a spy.

Five or six years ago, Mr. Fumio Ogawa (the adopted son of Mr. Kozo Ogawa, who personally worked with Dr. Usui and headed a

Reiki center) told us that Reiki practitioners had to move frequently during the war to avoid suspicion of belonging to the peace movement—which would have resulted in immediate execution.

Because the Reiki groups in Japan were either very small or highly secretive, they did not expand much through the years, and most groups ceased after World War II. Many of them disappeared with the death of their leader, and some of them changed the teachings to fit their own individual interests. Some of these groups even became something entirely different. I have heard that several contemporary Japanese mini-religions were started by some of Dr. Usui's students.

A large gap in Reiki history spans 1940 to the early 1980s. Mr. Fumio Ogawa mentioned that during the 1940s many Reiki schools existed all over the country. My father-in-law says that one of his fellow inmates in a Russian prisoner-of-war camp, a Japanese doctor, had talked to him about Reiki just after World War II. One of our students, a massage therapist and acupuncturist, told us that he had first heard about Reiki in the 1960s.

It is a well-known and somewhat-humorous fact of Japanese culture that techniques developed in Japan often need to be exported to the West and then reimported to become accepted by the Japanese people! One example is the art of macrobiotics, which was developed in Japan. It did not gain any support there until it had become a big hit in the United States and was then brought back to Japan. Aikido had the same fate, as did Shiatsu and Reiki. (In the following text, I will use the term "Western Reiki" when referring to the technique taught through Dr. Hayashi and Hawayo Takata and "Japanese Reiki" for the teachings of the Usui Reiki Ryoho Gakkai and other related Japanese groups.)

A great deal of the credit for reintroducing Reiki to Japan goes to Ms. Mieko Mitsui, a teacher of the Radiance Technique who brought Reiki back to her homeland in 1984. She taught Reiki One and Reiki Two classes in several Japanese cities and had several articles published in esoteric magazines. In one of the articles, she describes her meeting with Mr. Ogawa.[4] The article is the first documented meeting—complete with photographs—between Western Reiki and Japanese Reiki. Yet the results of that meeting were never discussed in public in the West.

Ms. Mitsui did not teach the Master level of Reiki in Japan. Eager practitioners who had learned Reiki One and Two came to Sapporo to do their teacher's training with Chetna and myself.

Within a few years, Western Reiki exploded throughout the country. Some of our students began teaching large classes in all major cities of Japan. By December 1999 Western Reiki had become a well-known technique in Japanese esoteric circles.

Several different schools of Western Reiki, based almost exclusively on either our students or our lineage, are now active in Japan. The biggest school is probably the one in Tokyo run by Mr. Toshitaka Mochizuki, author of the book Iyashi No Te,[3] who learned directly from us. He visited us twice with his employee, Mr. Takahashi, once in 1993 and once in 1998.

Other well-known Reiki teachers of our lineage are:

- Mr. Arupam Hitoshi Isono
- Mr. Fuminori Aoki, one of Mr. Mochizuki's students, author of the book *Healing the Reiki*, and president of the *Reiki One* association. *Reiki One* is the largest Reiki organization in Japan, not to be confused with the *Usui Reiki Ryoho Gakkai.*
- Mr. Doi, author of the book *Gendai No Reiki-Ho*
- Mr. Masaharu Ueno, author of the book *Shinden Reiki No Himitsu*
- Mr. Yoshio Tasaki, author of the book *Reiki Healing Jiten*
- Ms. Yukiko Utena, author of the book *Kyoi No Reiki Ryoho*

Japanese people are very skilled at taking a system of thought, a concept, a machine, a shoe, a technique, a song, or a religion into their own hands and changing it to something completely different. The end product is often much better than the original. Many of the aforementioned Reiki schools combine Western and Japanese Reiki.

Lineage has not been an important aspect of Western Reiki in Japan. Most Reiki practitioners/teachers do not know or care about where or when their teacher learned Reiki. However, it is not impolite to ask teachers about their lineage.

It has become a status symbol to be Japanese and teach Reiki in Western Reiki circles. However, don't be overly influenced by the nationality of a teacher. Instead, before you decide to study with any teacher, evaluate him or her the same way as you would appraise a teacher of your own culture.

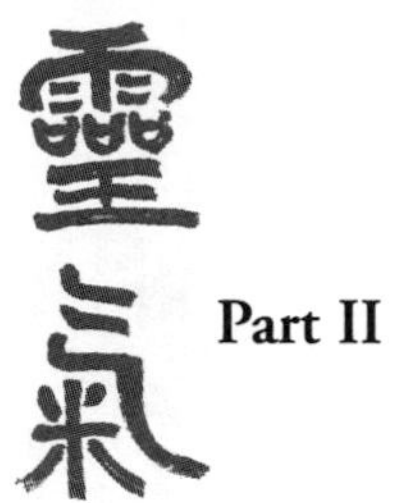

Part II

REIKI ENERGY BASICS

鬼神もなかすものは世の中の
人のこころのまことなりけり

: 37 ***Sincerity***
Of the human heart
In this world
Makes even a wrathful deity
Cry

CHAPTER 6

The Meaning of the Reiki Character

—by Walter Lübeck—

Much has been written and discussed about the mysterious symbols and mantras of the 2nd and 3rd Reiki Degrees, as well as the secrets that are concealed in them and the deeper understanding of the Reiki path that can be achieved by working with them. It is certainly correct that the "tool box"—the symbols and their mantras—of the Usui System of Natural Healing contains some important statements about the method.

A secret is best hidden within something apparent.

On the other hand, there is a central symbol that almost every friend of Reiki has already seen. It appears almost everywhere that Reiki can be found and *precisely* describes what Reiki is, how it works, where it comes from, and why it functions. This symbol is the character for Reiki. Oddly enough, there have been few publications or workshops about it up to now.

This chapter will extensively discuss the meaning of this interesting sign. It has many levels within its message, which reveal fascinating information about Reiki energy work and the Reiki philosophy, when taken as a whole. My involvement with this symbol has been of great help to me personally. It has been possible for me to work through many topics in a better way on the basis of the insights gained in this manner. My general understanding of energy work and spirituality has increased, making it possible for me to create an entire series of effective Rainbow Reiki techniques. Perhaps the involvement with the Reiki symbol will also help you advance on your path.

Today, people like to use the Japanese Reiki symbol for advertising, magazine articles, book titles, letterheads, posters, and business cards. It appears in publication in two variations.

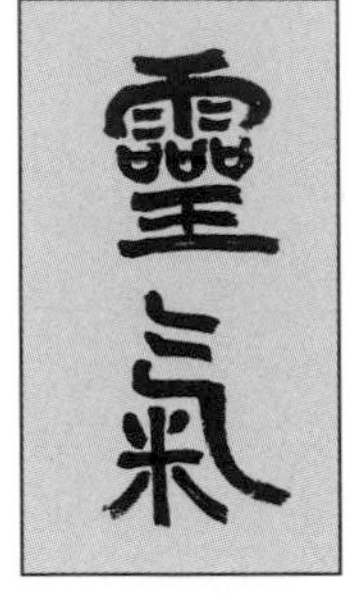

Picture 1
The old character for Reiki

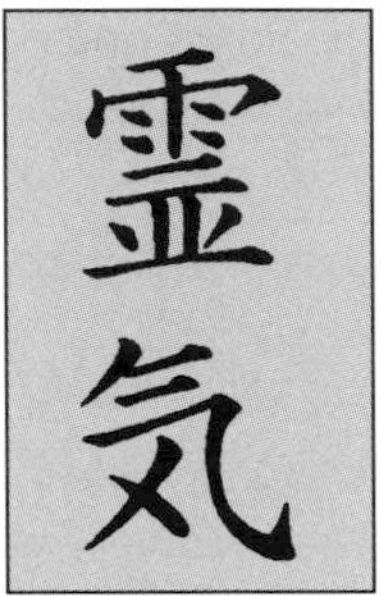

Picture 2
The new character for Reiki

The first version (picture 1) is an older, more original depiction that will be discussed extensively in this chapter. Although this is not the oldest way of writing, it still shows the individual components that give it meaning. Analyzing these components can lead to a deeper understanding of Reiki. The second version (picture 2) was developed within the scope of a spelling reform. It isn't possible to do much research work with this character since its parts are no longer in their original form. As a result, the inner message, especially of the upper portion, which stands for Rei or "spiritual," can no longer be understood clearly. Yet, this character is still the correct term for Reiki. It just contains too little of the explainable components.

So both signs are correct in the sense of expressing the word "Reiki" properly in writing. However, if we desire to more closely research the meaning of Reiki, we should prefer the original version since it can be more easily interpreted.

A little insight into history is important at this point: The Japanese characters were developed from the Chinese. In many respects, China had the function of a cultural and religious role model for Japan through the centuries. However, even in ancient times the Japanese tended to absorb influences from other cultures and adapt them to create their own special qualities.

In the Chinese language, the Japanese Reiki was called Ling Qi. To my knowledge, the first time it was mentioned in writing was in a treatise written around 300 B.C. by the Confucian philosopher Mencius (Mong Dsi). In this treatise, he complained that so many meditations were done in the monasteries with the goal of attaining worldly advantages: The truly meaningful aspect, the work in the sense of a personal opening of the human being to the divine by using Ling Qi, was neglected. It appears that every age has these kinds of problems.

An Analysis of the Reiki Character

In order to understand exactly what Reiki means, we must divide the respective character into its individual components. It is important to trace the way they are written and the meaning of these aspects back into history—to look at their roots.

Let's first look at the symbol for Ki ("Ki"—the modern way of writing it):

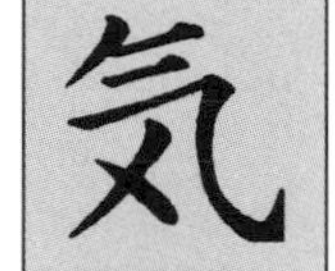

Picture 3

Picture 3 shows a calligraphy, which also plays a role in many other forms of subtle energy work, meditation, and medicine. The term Ki is used today in Japan in hundreds of compound words. There is even a Ki Lexicon that only lists expressions that contain Ki. Among other things, people in Japan understand Ki to be the following: spirit, soul, heart, intention, mood, temperament, and/or atmosphere (in the sense of a quality that surrounds a person, play, or work of art or prevails in a room).

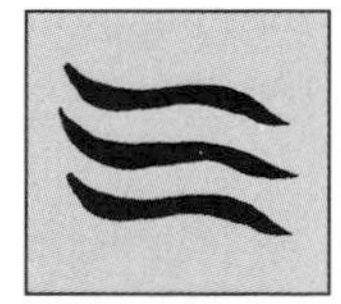

Picture 4

In its most original, oldest form, the upper portion—without the slanted cross—means "clouds." This can be interpreted as water that has been practically transformed in the spiritual sense and rises to the heavens. A further level of meaning is related to "praying" and "begging" (picture 4).

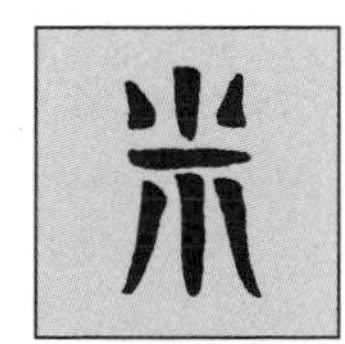

Picture 5

Later, a character for "rice" was added. Rice has been China's most essential food since ancient times and expresses the quality of the Chi that nourishes the body, mind, and soul (picture 5).

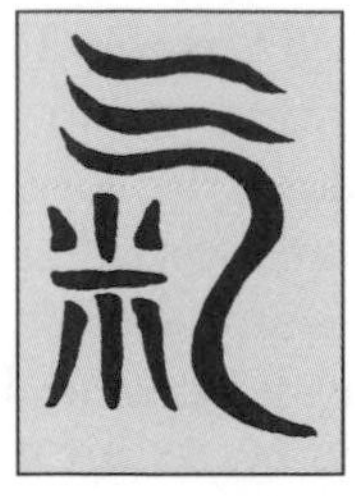

Picture 6

Accordingly, this is a very old version of the character for Ki (picture 6).

There are additional versions of the character for Chi in ancient China that are hardly used today. Picture 4 is therefore used as Ki in a number of variations and symbolizes cloud-like vapor. Incidentally, this has an interesting parallel to the extensive research by the great Austrian scientist Baron von Reichenbach. In the 19th Century, he carried out numerous experiments with medially talented people on the perception of various forms of life energy, which he called "Od." He discovered that this power was frequently perceived as a fine fog. English mediums have also reported similar observations. This old way of writing the Ki symbol basically represents something spiritual and energetically abstract that is separated from the material level or sent out in the form of a field and rises to the heavens, to the creative force.

As we all know, vapor rising from the earth leads to the formation of clouds and ultimately to rain. The rain returns to the earth, the material realm, to nourish it. The correlation of the character's meaning with prayer, ritual, and magical acts is clearly recognizable.

A statement from the Chinese classic Lei-zi (Lia Dsi), which was written in the period of the Quarreling Kingdom (475-221 B.C.) contributes important information to the meaning of the symbol for the vital force: "...What is spiritual, is part of the heavens. What is physical, is part of the earth. What belongs to heaven is pure and fleeting. What belongs to the earth is turbid and sticky. When the spirit leaves the form, both return to their true nature.[10]

This means that life ends when the soul belonging to heaven, the essence of a human being's spiritual nature, detaches from its material form, the body. On the other hand, there is the less drastic experience mentioned above. Here parts of the soul may rise to the heavens like vapor that has been freed from the bonds of its material connectedness through the warmth of the sun. It can rise from the ground to the bright expanse of the heavens, back to its origin in order to seek counsel and refresh itself in the source of life. Then, it will be strengthened and empowered to have an influence according to the wishes of the creative force in order to shape and regenerate life on the material level in a spiritual way.

The conditions required for this to occur are described in another Chinese book of wisdom, the *I Ching* (Book of Changes), in Chapter 11 with the title of "Peace." It involves placing the feminine, material, and yin *above* the masculine, spiritual, and yang in order to shape the life process constructively for all participants. Translated into the practice, this means that the spiritual perceptions and experiences must absolutely be turned into something that is useful in everyday life and that the body with its feelings, desires, and senses must be turned into a temple of the creative force. Then the divine within the human realm can be brought to life. This is practically the foundation of Indian Tantra, the art and science of using the body's sensuality and ability to feel pleasure for the purpose of spiritual experiences and personality development.

The opposite of what has been described in the last paragraph can be found in Chapter 12 of the *I Ching*, "Stagnation." This is symbolically depicted by the spiritual, masculine yang being placed above the material, feminine yin. Both of them no longer enter into a relationship with each other because the natural direction of the yang's movement tends upward, to the heavens, and the natural direction of the yin's movement tends downward, to the earth. Seen in practical terms, this means that spiritual experiences and perceptions are considered as an end in themselves and carefully kept away from everyday life while the energies and desires of the body are simultaneously lived without a connection to spiritual purposes. This can also be seen as an end in itself.

Here is an example of this situation: The partnership between a man and woman can be a spiritual path for both when the man strives to perceive, accept, and live the divine within himself while honoring and loving his wife as a goddess and when she strives to perceive, accept, and live the divine within herself while honoring and loving her husband as a god. This is the peace (described in Chapter 11 of the *I Ching*) that allows everything to thrive in love and joy. It radiates from such a couple in the form of a pleasant power, which has made the holy marriage into its life principle. However, if the partnership is designed in such a way that the husband looks down upon his wife because she is different than he is and she is disappointed with him because he is different than she is, with both considering their life together as nothing more than a formality with no deeper meaning, then the strife described in Chapter 12 of the *I Ching* will occur.

Additional Ways of Writing the Ki Character

One more ancient way of writing the character for Ki consists of connecting the upper portion of the character from picture 1, without the slanted cross added below, with the character for "fire" or for "breath and fire."

The meaning of this variation is that fire, which is related to the fulfillment of the personal, spiritual task in life according to Chinese mysticism, is called "duty" by Mencius (see below). This duty allows the divine center of human nature to become the determining portion of the individual over time. This process is explained in Chapter 30 of the *I Ching*, "Brightness." Only when we open our hearts for a spiritual task in the material world and become the bearer and steward of the spiritual light, the divine flame, will we become messengers of God. This cannot be accomplished with a formally practiced technique, but only through a deeply spiritual orientation in our way of living. The breath, which is included in some signs for Ki together with the fire, can be a powerful tool for freeing the body from blocks that impede the flow of the divine life forces, as every breath therapist knows. (Also see my statements on the relationship between the heart and the lungs in the chapter 20 on the whole body treatment on page 203 ff.) We can specifically direct our attention to the individual areas of the body and the organs through the breath. And wherever the attention is focused, the life force will flow more easily. The more freely the life force circulates within the body, the better it can free itself of waste materials and toxins, the higher and more spiritual its vibration will be. The higher its vibration, the more likely we will be to perceive our personal divinity and the divine light within ourselves. Then we can orient ourselves upon them as we walk our path in life.

Before I interpret the rest of the character, I would like to let Mencius* one of the foremost sages of ancient China, explain the meaning of the *Ki/Chi* concept:

"What we understand to be the life force *(Chi)* is something of the highest greatness, the highest strength. If it is nourished by the right things and not harmed, it will create the mediation between the invisible and the visible world. What we understand to be the life force belongs together with duty and with the meaning of life. Without these two, it can only atrophy. It is something that is created by the continual exercise of duty and not something that we can seize through one single act of duty." [10]

At another point in a didactic story, Mencius speaks of Chi as the soul, the center of our spiritual nature. It may help us better visualize this situation if we understand Chi to be a field that radiates from a human being's soul. If this field is weakened or blocked, then it can no longer keep the body in the state of liveliness. It becomes afflicted and ill, lacking in orientation and strength. The soul in this body is in the process of forgetting what it really is, where it comes from, and to where it will return. If the soul is now reminded of its true nature by the presence of the divine within itself, then it can again become oriented; its power and joy, trust in life, intuition and healing become strengthened.

In the famous Chinese classic by Chuang-Tzu "The True Book of the Southern Land of Blossoms", which was written around the 4th Century B.C., the following is said about Chi: "Human beings are born through the gathering of strength (Chi).** Life consists of

---

* Master Meng, also known under names like Meng-Tse or Mong Dsi was one of the most important students of the great Confucius. He lived from about 372-289 B.C.

** *What* causes the strength (Chi) to be gathered? It must be supplemented by "Rei", the Chinese "Ling".

strength (Chi). When Chi is dispersed, life ends. There is only one life force in the universe."

At another point in this work, Mencius describes that Chi, the life force, is created from the transformations of yin and yang.

Summary of the Esoteric Meaning of the Term Ki/Chi

Here are two valid interpretations of this complex term: Through a solar, "hot" force, an esthetic, nourishing quality that ascends to the heavens (to divinity) is released from matter. Or: By adding a large amount of energy to matter, the spiritual/divine components within it are strengthened. Even today, this principle is successfully applied in Taoist Yoga, in Indian Tantra, as well as Eastern and Western alchemy—and in Reiki.

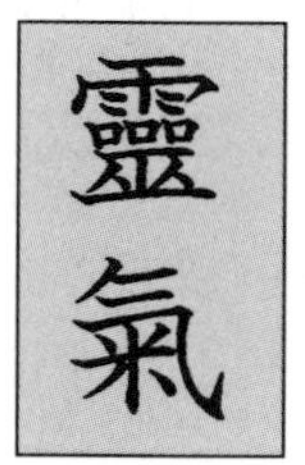

Picture 7

How does the "Ki" connect with the "Rei"?

The symbol "Rei" is written in an old form like this: Translated literally, it means: "spirit that is not defined qualitatively" or even "spiritual." In terms of the actual meaning, it can be translated as: "the secret meaning," as well as "the hidden force" (picture 7).

If we add the older layers of meaning found in the Chinese Ling to further clarify it, more detailed information results. The term was used in ancient China in such areas as Tantric-Buddhist and Taoist circles within the scope of energy work and meditation. This is similar to what I heard in a workshop on a certain method of Qi Gong by way of explanation: "If...this method is carried out, the spirit will become perfectly calm; this is called 'perfect' because it surpasses every type of earthly peace, even the repose of death. From this calm, the light (of the mind) crystallizes for enlightenment, the spiritual quality (*Ling*) of which generally penetrates the entire being of the meditator and his or her natural drives in the spiritual sense."

An archaic meaning from the era of the Taoist philosophy's development clearly enters the area of shamanism. "Rei" (Chinese: *Ling*) can be translated here as "rain-making." The upper portion of the symbol represents "rain." (picture 8). The middle part (picture 9)

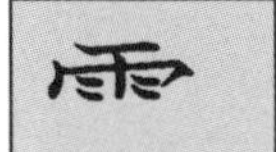
Picture 8

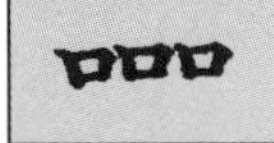
Picture 9

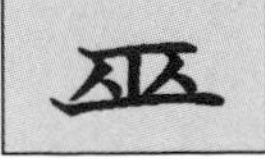
Picture 10

stands for three opened mouths and the lower section (picture 10) means "sorcerer" or "shaman."

To make this literal translation somewhat easier to understand, it can be interpreted like this: The shaman aligns the three parts of his being: the body (inner child), the mind (middle/rational "conscious" self), and the soul (higher self)—with their desire for a mutual goal, the rain. This feat requires the power of love, which wants to support truth, beauty, and kindness, as well as the receptiveness of the individual parts of the personal self. It also includes the desire to improve our own situation and that of the people around us. As already described above in the explanation of the term *Ki*, "rain" can be understood as the effect of the divine on a human being's expanded personal spiritual field. On the basis of this context, the Rainbow Reiki technique of providing an angel (as a representative of the creative force) with a distant Reiki treatment—as a sacrifice—will evoke a strong healing power from it in return. This can then have an effect in the material world through the person who sent the distance Reiki in the form of a Rainbow Reiki essence, for example.[11]

The trinity that manifests itself, such as saying a mantra three times in order to activate a Reiki symbol during a distance treatment, is an essential component of many forms of energy work today.

The divine is frequently also depicted in the form of a trinity.

In the classical Chinese texts, *Ling* continues to be seen as the constellating force that forms and moves the material structures according to the directions of the spiritual realm—in conjunction with *Ki*. *Ling* is generally the message without someone to deliver it, the letter without a stamp.

Although continuing involvement with these explanations of the Reiki symbol requires a certain amount of work, it can open up fascinating new insights.

CHAPTER 7

A Japanese System for Describing the Life Energies

—by Walter Lübeck—

Through my involvement with the traditional Asian healing arts and macrobiotics, founded by the Japanese George Ohsawa, I came across a very useful and informative Japanese system of classifying life energies at the beginning of the 1990s. This system closed an important gap in the information available to me. I couldn't imagine that Reiki was practically created "from nothing" by Mikao Usui. Whatever human beings develop always has its roots in the work, experience, and perceptions of other people. Consequently, there must also have been a certain type of environment from which Mikao Usui developed his Reiki System of Natural Healing. I found it particularly interesting to discover how much easier it is to understand Reiki itself through the description of the functions and features of other types of life energy, which form a system together with Reiki.

The life-energy system explained in this chapter is partially borrowed from the Chinese model of the Five Elements. It's no wonder that many of the spiritual ideas that are considered "original Japanese" today comes from China for the most part.

A significant origin of the system is certainly the primal, shamanically oriented Chinese Taoism. The important correlations of shamanism with Reiki have been discussed in the previous section.

Before we directly examine the "new" old Japanese system of vital energies, here are a few basic remarks about the concept of Ki.

In the Japanese language, "Ki" is considered the general term for all of the life energies. It is the Japanese version of the Chinese term Chi, with which we are familiar from Tai Chi Chuan, Qi* Gong,

* "Qi" is a synonim for "Chi" in the written language, according to an alternative transcription.

and Traditional Chinese Medicine. Moreover, there is an analogy between Ki and the concept of *Prana* from Eastern Indian philosophy. But Ki is not, as often claimed, the same as the type of vital force discovered by Wilhelm Reich, which he called *Orgon*. Because of the limited space available, it isn't possible to explain all of the differences. But the writings of Wilhelm Reich are certainly worth exploring. They contain detailed descriptions of orgon's special qualities that can be compared with the characteristics of Chi explained in this book and many writings on Traditional Chinese Medicine. This will make the differences in the concepts easy to understand.

Orgon is *one* expression of the life energy, but it is not a general term for the various types of subtle vital forces like Chi or Ki or Prana. This differentiation is important since the laws that apply to orgon are often applied to all types of Ki—but this does not function in the practice.

Speaking quite generally, life energies have certain characteristics that can be primarily observed in their synergetic interaction. This includes their mutual appearance with certain electromagnetic fields, their peculiarity of making independently acting organic systems possible and counteracting entropy, as well as the various ways of permitting these systems to strive for unity and reproduction.

Ki circulates in the human body in the form of various qualities that build upon each other.

1. Kekki
2. Shioke
3. Mizuke
4. Kuki
5. Denki
6. Jiki
7. Reiki

Consequently, the energy form called *Kekki*, listed in the following text under no.1 is that with the greatest power but with a very minor ability to organize.

The energy form listed under no.7 *(Reiki)* has the greatest ability to organize the flow of energy in the mind and body; but at the same time, it is hardly capable of having a *direct* effect. The last energy form listed here is therefore a type of control program, making sure that everything required within the human system is done with the right forces, in the proper proportion, at the appropriate time, in the most suitable rhythm, and in the most meaningful manner. The other energies between 1 and 7 exercise various functions in the interplay with each other, as described in the following.

It is certainly also important to know that energy organs—such as those familiar to us from the chakras of Indian yoga—will not be described here. Instead, these are energy qualities with unique characteristics. The forces occur in every energy organ of a being. However, they are most densely concentrated in the function bearer that is closest to them. Function bearers are for example the energy organs described in the previous sentence.

The Characteristics of the Seven Basic Life Energies

1. Kekki

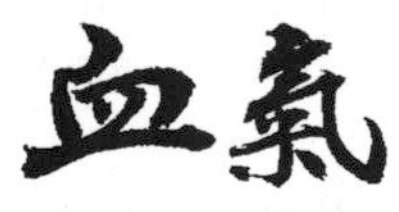

The form of Ki that provides a living being with nourishing strength, which is called *Kekki* in Japanese. *Kek* is derived from the word *Ketsu*, which means "blood" in translation. Consequently, *Kekki* is the "Ki of the blood," which is closely connected with the energy organ of the **1st chakra**, located at the end of the spine (coccyx). *Kekki* is used by the cells in order to maintain their substance and have energy to take action. This energy quality is created when, for example, an individual participates in the eternal flow of nourishing and being nourished during the exchange, feeding, and encounter with other earthly beings. *Kekki* is the coarsest and least structured energy quality in the body. It is therefore the easiest energy for the higher organizing forces to use in nourishing specific structures. *Kekki* is something like the clay from which any number of bricks can be formed, baked, and used to construct buildings. When *Kekki* is firmly integrated into a process in a certain way, it transforms into a different form of energy.

Kekki, the vital force, needs an opportunity to gather and to be the nourishment for something in order to fulfill its task within the scope of the Creation. It can't do it alone. When fulfilling this function, it receives help from the following energy quality.

2. Shioke

塩氣 This is the form of Ki that gives the body the structure in which the vitality (*Kekki*) can gather and have an effect. It helps it to "stay together" and not fall apart, even under strain, because there are enough reserves stored in the structure. It has the will and the steadfastness to continue its own existence and is called *Shioke* in Japanese. This word can be translated as the "Ki of the salt" or the "Ki of the minerals"*. *Shioke* is a structure equipped with connective power; it is the from in which *Kekki* is held for a time, which may correspond with the life span of a being or a cell. In this way, it creates the existence of the individual. This human force field is created when individuals recognize that their earthly embodiment basically has a purpose. Something that does not want to fulfill a purpose doesn't need a structure that is suitable for fulfilling a purpose. This means accepting our own earthly existence as a significant and lasting opportunity for experiencing and satisfying our own needs.

Shioke also represents the constitution of human beings, our fundamental possibilities of self-realization, and naturally also our boundaries. If *Shioke* is destroyed in a violent manner, the *Kekki* contained within it is free to leave it and nourish another *Shioke*, allowing it to function. *Shioke* is practically the vessel in which *Kekki* is stored and the latter energy also fulfills a specific function. This function is determined in part by the vessel and in part by other forces.

In addition, *Shioke*—like *Kekki*—has a close relationship with the **1st chakra**. In order for *Shioke* to fulfill its function and translate the meaning of its existence into action, it requires relationships with other animated substances and other beings, especially those of the type it represents. Its various expressions are created by the more highly organized life forces.

---

* This can be compared to the qualities of common salt (sodium), which is called *natrium muriaticum* in classical homeopathy.

3. Mizuke

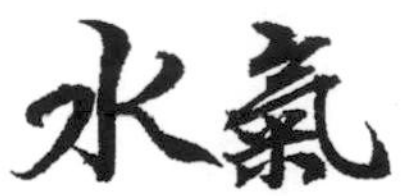

This is the expression of Ki that allows relationships to function as the basis of communication, therefore making it possible to dissolve the separation and experience of joy, playfulness, and a sense of security when we are together in a physical sense . It is called *Mizuke* and also makes many other important experiences possible. We could translate it as the "Ki of the water" or even the "Ki of liquids." *Mizuke* is the force of relationship, of "winning by giving in (devotion)." This life-energy quality is created when, for example, we accept that we are flowing along in the eternal interplay of developing and decaying, that each of us contributes to the perpetual dance of the creative forces in our own individual way. Among other things, *Mizuke* produces the fundamental emotional patterns of basic trust, desire, and the ability to be devoted to another person. It generally represents the original energy for all emotions. It is responsible for eroticism and sexuality, tenderness, and body consciousness. At the same time, it also makes it possible for us to take in nourishment of all kinds and supports the metabolism. *Mizuke* is closely associated with the energy organ of the **2nd chakra**, located just above the pubic bone in the lower abdomen. It is the force that brings together the *Kekki* bound within the various *Shioke* forms and creates structures from it. It makes the flow of forces from one form to another possible. Without *Mizuke*, the *Shioke* forms would remain isolated because they are caught within themselves, rigid and sluggish without any genuine movement. *Mizuke* probably corresponds with orgon, discovered by the ingenious Austrian scientist Wilhelm Reich.

In order for the many relationship possibilities to be filtered appropriately for individuals and their development and transformed into lasting, personally meaningful experiences, *Mizuke* must be specifically instructed by another force and practically shown the way.

4. Kuki

The form of Ki that helps create the appropriate relationships for the respective being with other parts of the Creation by producing boundaries, opening up in a specific way, shaping, and striving is called *Kuki*. The translation of this word is "Ki of the gases" or also "Ki of the air." *Kuki* is self-fulfillment: growing, becoming conscious of the self, and personally becoming in life in a meaningful way. This force field is manifested, for example, when we perceive and accept our individuality, involving it in the way we shape our lives. This quality of the Ki is closely associated with the **3rd chakra**, located beneath the sternum in the stomach area.

Among other things, *Kuki* supports the ability to think logically and break down nourishment. It is the power that a karate fighter uses to smash a concrete plate with bare fists; it is also an essential part of the powers that Philippine faith healers use to carry out operations with just their bare hands.

Kuki imparts the motivation for us to want to take our own path and experience who we are. Kuki also makes sure that we do not let ourselves become diverted from our own appropriate course under the influence of other people.

In order for growth and striving not to be at the cost of the surrounding world but realized for the benefit of the respective group, *Kuki* requires a force that helps it become oriented toward the true needs of an individual's personality and the beings with whom this person is *directly* connected. This means finding a mutual rhythm for dancing without everyone constantly stepping on each other's feet.

5. Denki

電氣

The form of Ki that lends us our striving, our relationship with the ego, and the urge to grow in a way considerate of others is called *Denki*. This can be translated as "Ki of the thunder." In this context, it is interesting that the power of the thunder in Hexagram No.51 of the Chinese book of wisdom and oracles, the *I Ching*, is said to have brought human beings into contact with the creative force. Although thunder initially causes us to be terrified and frightened, this cleansing experience can help us find the proper attitude toward worldly things and act in an ethical and moral manner.

This type of life energy is created within us when we accept that our growth should not happen at the cost of our own well-being or that of another person with whom we are involved. Among other things, *Denki* produces the emotional patterns of love, empathy, tolerance, and trust in God—but only under the condition that, under the influence of *Denki*, no other activities are done that could divert our attention.

We can understand this strange rule by remembering that thunder heals and purifies by frightening us. If we suppress this reaction by turning our attention to some sort of "harmless" occurrences, then *Denki* can't have a complete effect upon us. *Denki* gives life a socially organizing component that also greatly strengthens our drive for self-preservation—not because of fear, but through the power of loving what we are. This quality of the life energy also creates a natural fairness in the exchange with others, tolerance, and a well-meaning understanding of anything that is different.

In order for the considerate individual conduct produced by *Denki* to be controlled in such a way that our development does not come to a standstill by becoming completely integrated in the community and content with ourselves, an additional power quality is needed.

Denki is associated with the 4th **Chakra,** the heart-centre.

6. Jiki

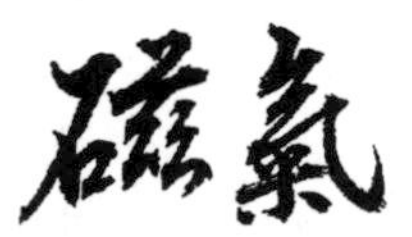

The form of Ki that helps us find the precisely appropriate complement to our own being in every situation, that presents us with our unlived shadow aspects in a way that we cannot overlook and simultaneously helps us develop our fallow talents through focusing attention on them, is called *Jiki*. This word can be translated as "magnetic power" or also "gathering force." This special force field is available to us when we accept the meaningful challenges and lasting relationships that are vital for our development in connection with responsibility. *Jiki* produces charisma and the structuring of our own form and surrounding world according to the true will, which has a divine source, and the three essential qualities of the creative force: It contains what is true, beautiful, and kind. *Jiki* therefore also represents the power of esthetics, art, and beauty in any form. It makes sure that "each pot gets the appropriate lid", which also increases the pressure in the pot when the heat is turned up since there is no escape from the situation. It's no coincidence if this metaphor makes you think of relationships. There are definitely correlations to be found here. *Jiki* shows the other energies and coordinate their expression, appropriate to the individual existence of the respective being. The magnetic expression of the life energy is connected with the **5th chakra**, which is located at the bottom of the neck above the chest.

In order for the forms of life energy described in the last six points to be appropriately attuned to each other in their effects and activated specifically in the sense of the life processes, there must be a controlling force on the highest level to provide for a stable flow equilibrium (homeostasis) in the entire system.

7. Reiki

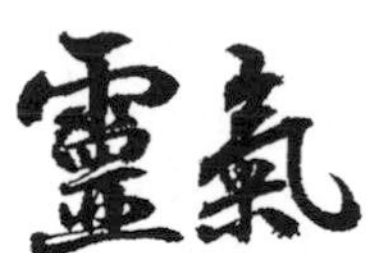

The form of Ki that organizes the correct synergetic application of all the subordinate forms of the life force in the holistic sense is called *Reiki*. This word can be translated as "soul force" or "spiritual power." It is this quality of the life energy that, in the material world, is closest to the divine creative force, the source of all life. It attunes the three archetypal partial personalities of the inner child, middle self, and higher self with each other so that all three remain connected with each other in one system instead of striving apart because of their differing characteristics.

- Reiki connects without binding.
- Reiki stimulates without overexciting.
- Reiki separates without creating isolation.
- Reiki calms without causing rigidity.
- Reiki directs our attention to life and the love in the heart
- Reiki creates clarity without a lack of involvement.
- Reiki wakes us up and supports the development of all types of latent potentials.

In my opinion, these are the essential types of effects of the universal life energy in its pure form. However, we still have to walk this path to reach it. In as far as Reiki receives adequate opportunity to do so, it will first make sure that cleansing and clarification take place as a precondition for the additional processes. In order to avoid self-poisoning despite thorough cleansing, we must decide to live in a different manner—healthier, more spiritual, and more individual. Reiki can't—and isn't allowed to—take over this act of willpower. The free will is a gift of the divine force. Mastering it is a holy duty—as is learning to use it in a way that is meaningful in terms of the whole of Creation.

Forms of the life energy that are higher and more uniform than Reiki cannot manifest themselves directly in the material world of separation.

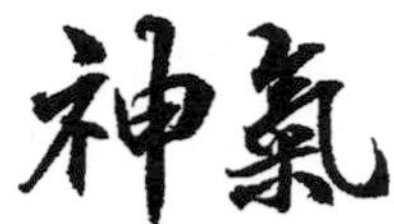

The *divine Ki*, from which everything is created and to which everything returns after the end of its material existence, is called *Shinki*. *Shinki* works outside of the material world above the 7th **chakra**, which is located about two to three fingers above the top of the head, through *Reiki*. Reiki is close enough to the principle of unity, as well as the principle of separation, to form an interface for the contact between the two. This function maintains the flow equilibrium of the streams of yin and yang. Summarized in one sentence, Reiki promotes all types of life processes.

Reiki is connected with the energy center of the forehead, the **6th chakra**. This can be found above the root of the nose between the eyebrows.

It should be mentioned once again that although the types of life energy described here have a close resonance with specific chakras, they are not to be understood as the energies of these chakras. These energies flow through the chakras. Subordinate forces, such as the meridians that we are familiar with from acupuncture, are then set into motion and certain types of behaviors are triggered. The various types of life energy explained in this chapter therefore represent the more primary qualities than the subsequent life energies that circulate directly in the main and secondary chakras, the organs, and the meridians.

CHAPTER 8

The Nature of Reiki Energy

—by William Lee Rand—

I became interested in metaphysics in high school and was fascinated by the idea that we have dormant abilities within us. The ability to enhance our creativity, to have more energy to sleep more soundly, to be telepathic and intuitive, and to communicate with spirits was very intriguing to me. But the one ability that was the most interesting was the ability to heal ourselves and others.

I grew up during the cold war and the threat of global nuclear destruction. At that time the whole world could have been destroyed in a half an hour, and it might have happened because of a computer error or a poor decision. This was frightening! Although this was the worst problem, many others existed as well. I felt that if we had dormant abilities within us, then perhaps they could be awakened and used to heal the problems of the world and make the earth a better place to live.

So I began reading all I could about spiritual abilities and metaphysics and was attracted to the Rosicrucian Order. I joined and began receiving their lessons. I was soon told that you shouldn't believe something simply because someone says it's true or because it's written in a book. They said people can say anything, whether it's true or not, and that a printing press will print whatever a person wants it to. And while we can evaluate the statements of others by looking at what they base their ideas on, the most important way of learning is by doing. The Rosicrucians said that the best way to learn about life and especially about metaphysics was from experience, to try things and form your own opinion about the metaphysical world by interacting with it and by having a direct conscious connection to metaphysical forces and energies. This was a powerful idea! I really found value in the ideas, because all my teachers up to that point simply said, "Just believe us. We're adults, and we know what we are talking about. Don't question what we say, but just believe us because we are right." Unfortunately, this seems to be what happens in most public schools; they don't encourage students to trust in their own inner authentic sense of direction. Instead, they demanded that students conform to what society states to be important. But the Rosicrucians said it was better to develop your own ability to decide what was useful and what was true and to learn about the world, both inner and outer by experiencing it.

So I decided I would learn all I could about metaphysics by doing the experiments they offered and by taking other training. Over the course of the next twenty years I proceeded to take a wide range of metaphysical and inner-development classes and courses. I would often study and practice a particular subject until I could begin offering sessions professionally to others. During that time I became a hypnotherapist, a past-life-regression therapist, an astrologer, a rebirther, an NLP Professional, and a tarot-card reader. While living in Hawaii, I studied and worked with a Kahuna for over a year.

As I learned each new subject, I found that my previous training and experience would add to my understanding of the new skills, thus broadening my comprehension. I found I could often create unique ways to apply the new skills that had not been thought of by those trained in only one area. As an example, I combined my understanding and experience with hypnosis, past-life-regression therapy, and NLP to create a powerful technique that allowed me to take clients back to the original cause of any problem or challenging situation and discover how they created the experience. Then, we would focus on learning the lesson, healing the cause, and transforming the issue into a positive quality.

In the course of my studies, I also learned about life force and the important role it plays in maintaining life. Life force, or Ki, is a subtle energy that surrounds and flows within all life. Ki keeps living entities alive and healthy. If the Ki is removed or greatly weakened in a living entity, it will soon die. All illness is caused by disturbances in the healthy flow of Ki within the subtle energy system. This metaphysical energy is present everywhere and has a wide spectrum of vibrations and levels of expression, depending on the kind of life and life processes it is supporting. Ki is a necessary energy for everything that exists, both living and nonliving, in the material world as well as in all spiritual worlds. In humans, a range of different vibrations of Ki are present in the aura and chakras. There is a very basic Ki which has to do with sustaining the physical body, a Ki is involved with our thoughts and feelings, and a higher Ki has to do with our spiritual experiences. Ki is the carrier of our intentions out into the world where they manifest and it is Ki directed by our minds that attracts to us all of our experiences. From this we can see that Ki plays a very important role in every aspect of life. Ki is an amazing subject, and a great deal can be written about it. But for our purpose in understanding the nature of Reiki energy, we need to focus on its activity within the human subtle-energy system.

I came across several exercises to develop Ki and use it for healing. The exercises usually involved meditation and breathing; when doing them, I could feel the buildup of Ki within my body and energy field and could move the energy around with my intention. I could also see it inside myself and feel the way it affected me. Ki usually created a very relaxing and pleasant feeling.

The Kahuna I worked with was a healer and could also generate and use Ki. The word "Kahuna" is derived from the Hawaiian words ka and Huna. Huna means "secret" and Kahuna means "Keeper of the Secret." The term is used because the Kahunas did not frequently pass their techniques on to others. Rather, they kept them in the family or in a very closely determined group, almost always of Hawaiian ancestry. The group usually had just one student to whom they gave all their knowledge. The training of this one student took place over many years, with the most important lessons being passed on just before the senior Kahuna died. The tradition eventually became more open, and I was very fortunate to have been given some of the Kahuna's teaching when I was with him.

In working with him, my understanding of Ki deepened, and it became even clearer that Ki is effected by the mind and can be directed by the mind. It can be sent to heal or help others, but it was also clear that it could be sent to cause problems for others and even to create illness. One of the Kahuna skills involved protecting people from negatively directed Ki sent by others. The Kahunas of Hawaii had become experts in the use of Ki. The basis of most of their work is using Ki in various ways to create a wide range of effects. I have also met many other healers and metaphysical people who had awareness of and skill in using Ki. They all reported that Ki can be built up in one's system and directed by the mind to heal oneself or others, and to do many other things.

Why People Get Sick

If Ki could only do good, then we would live in a very different world. But since Ki is effected by the mind, it can create both positive and negative results depending on the thought or intention directing it. Ki directed by the mind is responsible for both our good and bad health. It is the positive Ki, created and directed by the subconscious mind, that empowers all organs of the body and keeps them healthy. But the subconscious mind can also harbor negative thoughts; when the thoughts are about oneself, they influence personal Ki in a negative way. The negatively directed Ki will form around the organs of the body and in the chakras and aura, slow down the healthy activities of the body, and eventually create sickness. It is negative Ki that is responsible for creating disfunction and illness in the body. Healers can often see negative Ki as dark spots or clouds in or around the body that are obstructing the flow of healthy Ki. By removing the negative Ki, the healthy Ki is allowed to flow again and return the body to health.

Negative Ki can have a very simple charge of energy and be easy to remove, or have a more powerful charge and a more sophisticated programming and be more difficult to remove. It can be deceptive and act like it is healthy while possessing an underlying negative intention, or it can hide, making it difficult to detect. This is based on the thoughts that used to create it—thoughts coming from the person's subconscious mind or even conscious mind which combine with Ki and take action to effect the functioning of the body, the emotions and the mind. From this it can be seen how important it is to develop a positive self-image and to release all negative thoughts and feelings from our minds.

Throughout our lives, we are exposed to millions of thoughts and feelings from others. They affect our minds, depending on how receptive we are to them. When we are young, we are like an open book, and it is difficult for us to decide which thoughts and feelings to accept or reject. During the formative years, the foundation of our personalities is established, and we are usually influenced most strongly by our parents. We also receive programming from television, teachers at school, and other experiences. These beginning concepts become established in our subconscious mind, and this in turn forms a pattern of positive and negative Ki in our auras, chakras, and bodies. The pattern directly effects our health, as well as everything we do and experience.

Others can also place negative Ki in our energy fields. They sometimes do so unconsciously when they harbor dark negative thoughts toward us. The negative Ki will affect those of us who have a weakness in the aura or chakras. The negative energy is often called bad vibes and can have a temporary effect. It can also harm more permanently if the receiving person is weak or otherwise open to the negative energy and if it is directed in a more powerful and deliberate way.

Our minds and subtle energy fields are also affected by experiences from past lives. This effect, called karma, is carried into life in the aura when the soul first enters the physical body at birth. Through life, the past-life karma in the aura attracts experiences to us, which in turn strengthens the karmic charge in the aura, then eventually it can move into the chakras, and eventually into the physical body. As it works its way deeper into the energy system, the effects become more pronounced and, depending on whether it is positive or negative, it can affect us in different ways, attracting good fortune or bad and also having a similar range of effects on our health. This is the basis of poor health and sickness.

Negative thoughts from ones own mind, or from past lives or that have been received from others, attracting or even generating negative Ki and affecting ones energy field by limiting healthy Ki, and restricting the functioning of the bodily organs. Healers heal by generating positive Ki and sending it to the area of the aura, chakras or body where the negative Ki is located, with the intention of transforming the negative Ki to positive or releasing and dissipating it. This allows the natural flow of positive Ki to take place. Regardless of the method involved, all processes of healing or personal and spiritual development involve releasing negatively directed Ki from a person's energy field, along with the negative thoughts and feelings that have created it. This is the primary process used by all shamans and healers all over the world. They employ a wide range of techniques to do this, but the purpose is the same. I learned this from personal experience working with Ki within myself and others and from the Hawaiian Kahuna and many other healers I have worked with.

Reiki Initiation: A Personal Experience

I received Reiki I in 1981 from Bethal Phaigh while I was living in Hawaii. It was a remarkable experience. When I first heard of Reiki, I wondered if it was real. I thought that the idea of Reiki and the attunement that went with it might be only a process of encouragement to instill confidence in the healing ability we already had rather than actually receiving the ability to use a new healing energy. So, remembering what the Rosicrucians had said about not believing something simply because someone says it is true. I decided that when I received the attunement, I would clear my mind and aura and witness what happened to see if it was just suggestion or if something really did take place energetically. During the attunement, I saw a new energy coming down through my crown chakra and then into my heart where it exploded out. I could actually see small chunks of something being blown out of my heart chakra as though it were being cleared of a block. I could also feel energy flowing into my hands. Then, after the attunements, I noticed a new energy flowing within myself. Because of this experience, I knew that Reiki was real and that the attunement had created an important improvement in my energy system.

When I began using Reiki, I realized right away that Reiki was remarkably different than the kind of Ki I was previously familiar with. Reiki seemed to have a higher vibration, and I noticed it did not need direction from my mind, but seemed to have a mind of its own. It would begin to flow without me doing any kind of exercise. I did not have to meditate or do breathing exercises and it seemed to flow all by itself whenever I placed my hands on someone or simply thought about it. It also did not make use of my own personal energy supply, but seemed to come from outside myself, from a seemingly unlimited supply. Sometimes it even began flowing all by itself. Often, I could observe it flowing through my arms and out my hands and sometimes through my aura. It was a very pleasant experience.

When I looked psychically at the energy, I could often see it as thousands of small particles of light, almost like corpuscles, filled with radiant Reiki energy flowing through me and out my hands. It was as though these Reiki corpuscles had a purpose and their own intelligence and were traveling through me to heal some part of myself or the person I was working with. When meditating on the Reiki energy I would often become filled with joy and be uplifted, often feeling that I was completely cared for and without a worry in the world. From these experiences, I knew that Reiki was something special. It was much more than the simple Ki I had previously learned to generate and move with my mind. This was an energy that came effortlessly and, rather than needing to be guided by my mind, it was being guided by a higher intelligence!

The special nature of Reiki energy has been continually demonstrated to me whenever I have used it, and others have frequently mentioned it to me as well. I became a Reiki master in 1989 and began teaching Reiki. At that time I had been working with two clairvoyant healers with remarkable abilities. They could each clearly see the aura and chakras, communicate with one's guides and higher self, see and communicate with angels and other spiritual beings, and analyze one's energy field in great detail. They could see and move negative Ki with their minds and heal from a distance. Their metaphysical diagnosis was always impressively accurate, and I would often be given a much deeper and more detailed understanding of my own energy state and what I needed to do to heal whenever I received a reading from them. They also had the ability to easily generate very strong Ki and use it to heal.

When I became a Reiki master, I offered them the training for free. They later told me that they had attended just to support me in my new work as they believed they already had highly developed healing abilities and did not think they would benefit by receiving Reiki. However, after the attunement, they both stated it had been a powerful spiritual experience and they had received a deep healing. Then, when they began using their new Reiki energy, they were even more pleasantly surprised. They said that Reiki was a new energy they had not experienced before. They remarked that it would begin flowing all by itself and did not require them to develop healing energy by meditating or through the use of their minds. They also said it seemed to have a mind of its own and had such a high frequency that it could go anywhere. It did not have to travel through the energy meridians of the body, but just went directly where it was needed, going through bone, muscle, and other tissues. Needless to say, they were very happy they had taken the class. Even though they were highly skilled healers, they felt the Reiki I training had noticeably improved their healing abilities!

The Special Healing Energy of Reiki

After teaching Reiki classes full time for over ten years and initiating over thirty-five hundred people, I have had the pleasure of working with many students who were already sensitive healers before taking Reiki training. The common response from the majority of this group, and especially from the most sensitive, is that Reiki has a different vibration than the healing energies they already were using. Taking the training had increased the strength of their healing energies and improved the quality of their treatments. All were happy they had taken Reiki training. Any healer, even one with powerful healing abilities, always seems to benefit from receiving the Reiki attunement.

So from this we can see that Reiki is a special healing energy that is much more than simple Ki. Reiki is Ki guided directly by the higher power, also known as. God, the Supreme Being, The Universe, The Universal Mind, All That Is, Jehovah, Krishna, Buddha, The Great Spirit, etc.

Because Reiki is guided by the higher power, it knows exactly what to do to help the person heal and it knows exactly where negative Ki exists in the person's subtle energy system. Reiki will usually flow to these areas where it changes the vibration of negative Ki. This is usually done by raising the vibration until the negative Ki cannot hold on to the area it is attached to and is released. Other times, the negative Ki may be reprogrammed by the Reiki energy and transformed into positive Ki which restores and maintains health. When the body is weak, from a healing crisis or from an extended illness, Reiki can provide the body with a very nurturing supply of Ki that helps the organs return to healthy functioning. On a deeper level, Reiki can and often does reprogram the person's subconscious mind, releasing negative thoughts, feelings, and memories and even balancing karma, all of which are responsible for creating negative Ki, thus healing at the level of cause and creating a permanent healing!

Because Reiki is guided by the higher power, it cannot do harm and always works for the positive benefit of the client. It is a very simple technique to learn and use and can be easily learned in a weekend class. Benefits of a treatment range from simple relaxation and feelings of well being to the miraculous. Occasionally, amazing healings come from people who have just taken their first class! Remarkably, Reiki does not take special ability or years of practice. Anyone can learn it in a day or two and experience effective results immediately!

We live in a world where a full range of experience can take place from the very positive to the very negative. People sometimes have joyful experiences and are filled with love, peace and happiness, and at other times can be unhappy with varying degrees of pain, sadness, and despair. Others seem to live in a relatively neutral and gray sort of world, half asleep and not feeling much of anything. This range of personal experience is taking place because of the way we use our free will. Because we have limited awareness and understanding, we do not always make the best choices. Sometimes we act out of fear, and often our selfish ego centered side takes over and begins directing our thoughts, feelings and actions. When this happens, we move away from wholeness and create imbalances and distress that have a negative effect on ourselves and those around us. At other times we may allow our lives to be directed by our spiritual core and then healing takes place; our lives move toward harmony, joy and peace. So, we live in a world that seems to see/saw back and forth between wholeness and discord.

While this is taking place for most of us, there is another part of the universe, which is really just a state of mind, where this see/saw effect does not take place and only wholeness, harmony, peace, love, and joy exist there. All the beings here have surrendered completely to the higher power that directs their minds and actions. The place is also filled with many different kinds of Ki, also directed by the higher power. This higher dimension has been recognized by every religion and spiritual path. Young children are aware of it, and many adults glimpse it from time to time. It is also a state of consciousness that many have entered briefly, and a few have entered permanently even while still in the physical body. This higher dimension is where Reiki energy comes from, where all is at one with the higher power.

The great beauty and value of Reiki is that it connects us to the part of the universe where all is guided by the wisdom, love, and peace. When we receive a Reiki treatment, we get a taste of the higher dimension; at the same time, Reiki points us toward a greater experience. If we listen closely to the energy, the consciousness of Reiki, we will realize that it is offering the possibility that this higher dimension could be our continuous and unending reality. Every aspect of our mind, our lives, our entire being, could be continually surrounded and guided by the love, beauty, wisdom, peace, and grace of the higher power. It is the creation of this state of consciousness within each person that is the deeper intention of Reiki. As we discover this deeper intention for ourselves and open more and more to it, our lives will be transformed.

CHAPTER 9

A Scientific Explanation of Reiki Energy

—by William Lee Rand—

Some aspects of healing work are beginning to be understood from scientific standpoint. The most important standpoint for formulating a theory of how Reiki involves the electromagnetic fields generated by all living things. James Oschman, Ph. D. explains the fascinating subject in his recent book, "Energy Medicine, the Scientific Basis." [21]

It has been known for some time that electric currents flow through the body. These currents flow through the nervous system and are one of the ways the body regulates itself. The nervous system is connected to every organ and tissue in the body and signals flow through it from the brain to regulate all bodily activities.

Electric currents also flow from the heart through the circulatory system made possible by the saline solution of the blood, providing an additional pathway for electrical currents to flow. Over 50,000 miles of blood vessels allow the "heart electricity" to flow to every part of the body.

Electric currents flow in and between all the cells of the body. Many of the body's cells actually contain liquid crystals. The living crystals are in cell membranes, in the myelin sheathes of nerves, and in many other locations.[12] All crystals produce piezoelectric effects when pressure is placed on them. The liquid crystals in the body are therefore continuously generating electric currents. The currents are often coherent, meaning that like a laser the frequencies are all in step within a given area. The laser-like vibrations can travel within the body and also radiate into the environment. This brings to mind the potential healing effects of drumming. As the percussive pressures of the drumbeat interact with the tissues of the body, rhythmic electric currents and fields are created, affecting the biological activity of the tissues.

A second nervous system exists, called the perineurium, which is composed of a layer of connective tissue that surrounds the nervous system. Robert O. Becker described it in a series of articles.[13] More than half the cells in the brain are perineural cells. The perineurium operates on direct current. It is controlled by brain waves and is directly involved in the healing process. When any part of the body is injured, the perinerual system generates an electrical potential at the injury site that alerts the body to the injury. Through the use of these electrical potentials, the perinerual system directs repair cells to the site, such as white blood cells, fibroblasts, and mobile skin cells. The electrical potential changes as the injury heals. The perineural system is also very sensitive and responsive to exterior magnetic fields.

Whenever you have an electric current flowing through a conductor, a magnetic field surrounds the conductor. The electric currents flowing in human beings generate magnetic fields called biomagnetic fields that penetrate and surround the human body. Sensitive magnetometers have measured the biomagnetic fields. A device called a SQUID (Super Conducting Quantum Interference Device) was used by Dr. John Zimmerman at the University of Colorado School of Medicine in Denver to measure the biomagnetic fields of many parts of the body, including the brain, the heart, and many of the organs. The biomagnetic readings are becoming useful in understanding how the body works and in diagnosing illness.[14]

The heart has the strongest biomagnetic field and has been measured to a distance of 15 feet. The brain and all the organs of the body have their own biomagnetic fields surrounding them. The fields pulsate at various frequencies and interact with each other. An organ will have a specific frequency when it is healthy and will move away from this healthy frequency when it is not. The sum of all the biomagnetic fields forms a large aggregate biomagnetic field that surrounds the body. It is of course similar to what we call the aura. Therefore, the biomagnetic field may be one of the main components of the aura, although there may be other aspects to it as well.

The fields interact with other fields near the body, including the fields of other people. The principle is called induction and means that one magnetic field can have an effect on another, inducing changes in the field as well as changing the strength and frequency of the electric currents flowing in its conductor. So, the biomagnetic field of one person has an effect on the biomagnetic field of another.[15] The effect can influence the well-being of each person as well as the functioning of the organs and tissues. This gives real meaning to the term "magnetic personality." It is also the scientific basis for one person having a therapeutic effect on another.

So, from a scientific standpoint, a person's being does not stop at the skin, but extents out into the surrounding space. On a level of personal experience, we know it to be true, as we have all felt the presence of others. Now it has been proven and explained scientifically.

The hands also have biomagnetic fields surrounding them. The biomagnetic fields of healers hands have been measured while healing and were found to be much stronger than those of nonhealers. A simple magnetometer was used consisting of two coils of 80,000 turns each and was hooked to an amplifier. Healers' hands had a field strength of 0.002 gauss, which is one thousand times stronger than any other field emitted from the body.[16] The field pulsed at a variable frequency between 0.3 and 30 Hz, with most of the energy in the 7-8 Hz range.

The healing energy in the hands is at least partially generated by the perineural system. The system surrounds the nerves and is a pathway for direct electric currents. The currents are modulated by brain waves, which in turn are controlled by the thalamus.[17]

Other forms of energy besides biomagnetism may come from the hands and have a therapeutic effect. Some evidence suggests that infrared rays, microwaves, and other forms of photon emission come from healers hands and that biological systems are responsive to them.

When a person is sick, one or more of the organs of the sick person's body will have biomagnetic frequencies not in the healthy range for those organs. Herbert Fröhlich, a researcher who has discovered many interesting aspects about the body's biomagnetic fields, explains the process: "An assembly of cells, as in a tissue or organ, will have certain collective frequencies that regulate important processes, such as cell division. Normally these control frequencies will be very stable. If, for some reason, a cell shifts its frequency, entraining signals from neighboring cells will tend to reinstall the correct frequency. However, if a sufficient number of cells get out of step, the strength of the system's collective vibrations can decrease to the point where stability is lost. Loss of coherence can lead to disease or disorder."[18] This concurs with the metaphysical concept that illness starts first in the aura or biomagnetic field before developing in the physical body.

When a healer places her hands near a sick organ and begins to heal, the biomagnetic field emitted from the healers hands becomes much stronger than that emitted by the sick organ. The frequency of the biomagnetic field of the healer's hands also begins pulsing at the healthy frequencies needed by the organ. Because the healer's biomagnetic field is much stronger than the sick organ, it induces the healthy frequencies into the field of the sick organ, causing it to adjust its frequencies back into the healthy range. The adjustment in turn affects the electrical currents flowing in the cells and nervous system within and around the organ, as well as it's biological processes, and healing takes place.

Some of the healing frequencies for various tissues of the body have been researched. Nerves heal at a frequency of 2 Hz, bone at 7 Hz, ligaments at 10 Hz and capillaries at 15 Hz.[19]

The process can also work in the opposite direction when a healer is scanning or attempting to find areas of distress in a patient's biomagnetic field. During this process, the healer slowly moves one or both hands a few inches above the body, paying attention to sensations in the palm of their hand (s. page 162 *Byosen*). The patient's field induces changes in the field of the healer's hands that the healer can feel. The healer is thus able to locate areas of distress in the patient's biomagnetic field.

One of the unique qualities of Reiki is that the ability to do it comes from an attunement. Also, Reiki doesn't have to be guided by the conscious mind of the healer, but directs itself and does not use the healer's own personal energy. So, with the foregoing theories in mind, how might the Reiki attunement and treatments work? The attunement could awaken an innate aspect within each of us that has a higher level of intelligence concerning wholeness, well-being, and healing. Because the intelligence resides outside our conscious minds, it would be appropriate to say that the intelligence comes from a superconscious source within us. Also, the fact that it does not draw on one's energy indicates that the attunement activates an energy source different than the source of energy supplying our everyday needs. Therefore, Reiki validates the idea that we have hidden potential, dormant in most people but able to be awakened. The superconsciousness may then guide the functioning of the thalamus and the perineural nervous system to generate Reiki energy and direct it to the injured site through the healer's hands. Reiki energy may simply be a special mix of biomagnetic and other energies determined by the superconscious mind to be exactly what the part of the body where the hands are being placed needs in order to restart and complete the healing process.

Using these concepts, we can imagine that more powerful or effective kinds of healing may be possible if even higher aspects of the superconscious mind are called into use to formulate special combinations of energy frequencies and strengths to bring about healing more quickly and in more difficult cases. The healing might involve special combinations of love, compassion, and grace that provide greater encouragement for the injured part to let go of old patterns and return to health. The more powerful healing can be likened to an unusually skilled auto mechanic who, because of greater experience and understanding, is able to fix cars that other mechanics are not. As we increase our understanding and heal ourselves more deeply, our potential as healers will continue to awaken and enable us to contact higher aspects of the superconscious mind and develop even greater skill!

Biomagnetic fields decrease quickly in strength the farther you get from the source of the field. So, while the aforementioned theories can explain healing when the healer is in close proximity to the patient, how can distant healing be explained when a patient could be many miles away or even on the other side of the planet?

Scalar waves may be responsible for distant healing. When two magnetic fields are of exactly the same frequency and are exactly out of phase, they cancel each other out. The cancellation doesn't eliminate the effect of the fields, as the potentials are still there and they create what are called scalar waves. Scalar waves do not interact with electrons as magnetic fields do, but with atomic nuclei. They cannot be blocked by Faraday cages or other shielding and propagate to any distance without decreasing in strength. They also have been shown to effect biological tissue and can promote healing.[20] The waves may actually be the primary source of healing effects, rather than magnetic fields. According to Dr. James Oschman, "It is widely assumed that it is the electric and magnetic fields that interact with organisms, but some researchers suspect that scalar and potential waves actually underlie these effects." [21]

Even if the theories explain to a certain extent how healing works, one aspect of healing and spiritual work still remains a mystery. Biomagnetic fields and scalar waves are dependent on a physical body or other physical device to generate them. But many spiritual healers have direct experiences with higher beings that send healing. They do not have physical bodies. How is their healing energy generated? From a scientific understanding, how could they even exist? These questions are fertile ground for developing a deeper understanding of healing and of the nature of consciousness.

The living tissues of the body, being composed of molecules and atoms, are directly connected to and affected by all the forces of nature. It is only natural to assume that as living things evolved, the forces would become incorporated into the functioning of the body. This includes the known as well as unknown forces. By studying living things and especially ourselves, we are presented with the opportunity to understand even the deepest and most mysterious forces of the universe. It is likely that as science continues to study healing and the spiritual worlds, amazing discoveries will be made that will stretch our minds and bring about a transformation for life on our planet.

CHAPTER 10

The Meridians

—by Frank Arjava Petter—

In order to understand Dr. Usui's Japanese Reiki techniques more deeply, we must take a closer look at the Chinese system of meridians. In simple terms the meridians are energy pathways that supply our physical and subtle bodies with vital energy. If the energy flow is disturbed or disrupted, the result is sickness, disease, and, ultimately, death. The meridians run beneath the skin; the area where the meridians come close to the surface of the skin are, referred to as acupuncture points, acupressure points, or pressure points.

A vast amount of in-depth information on meridians is readily available in English, so it does not need to be discussed in great detail here. Anyone with a deeper interest in the subject can refer to the textbooks on acupuncture, Traditional Chinese Medicine, and Qi Gong or Tai Chi.[22, 23] Ultimately, it would be necessary to study with a licensed teacher to become proficient in one of the healing arts.

As a scholar of esoteric Buddhism, which came to Japan from China, Dr. Usui did not base his Reiki system on the Indian theory of the chakras or the Western system of the endocrine glands. Instead, he based it on Traditional Chinese Medicine and Qi Gong. You may be familiar with the twelve main meridians of the body. If not, you will most likely be surprised to find out that the way you may have been experiencing the movement of energy within your body is common knowledge in the East.

The illustrated meridians are listed here[32]:

Yin and Yang

The theory of yin and yang rules Chinese philosophy, as well as Traditional Chinese Medicine. The first mention of it is found in the Book of Changes, the *I Ching*, and it is the red thread that runs through thousands of years of Chinese literature. Yin and yang are

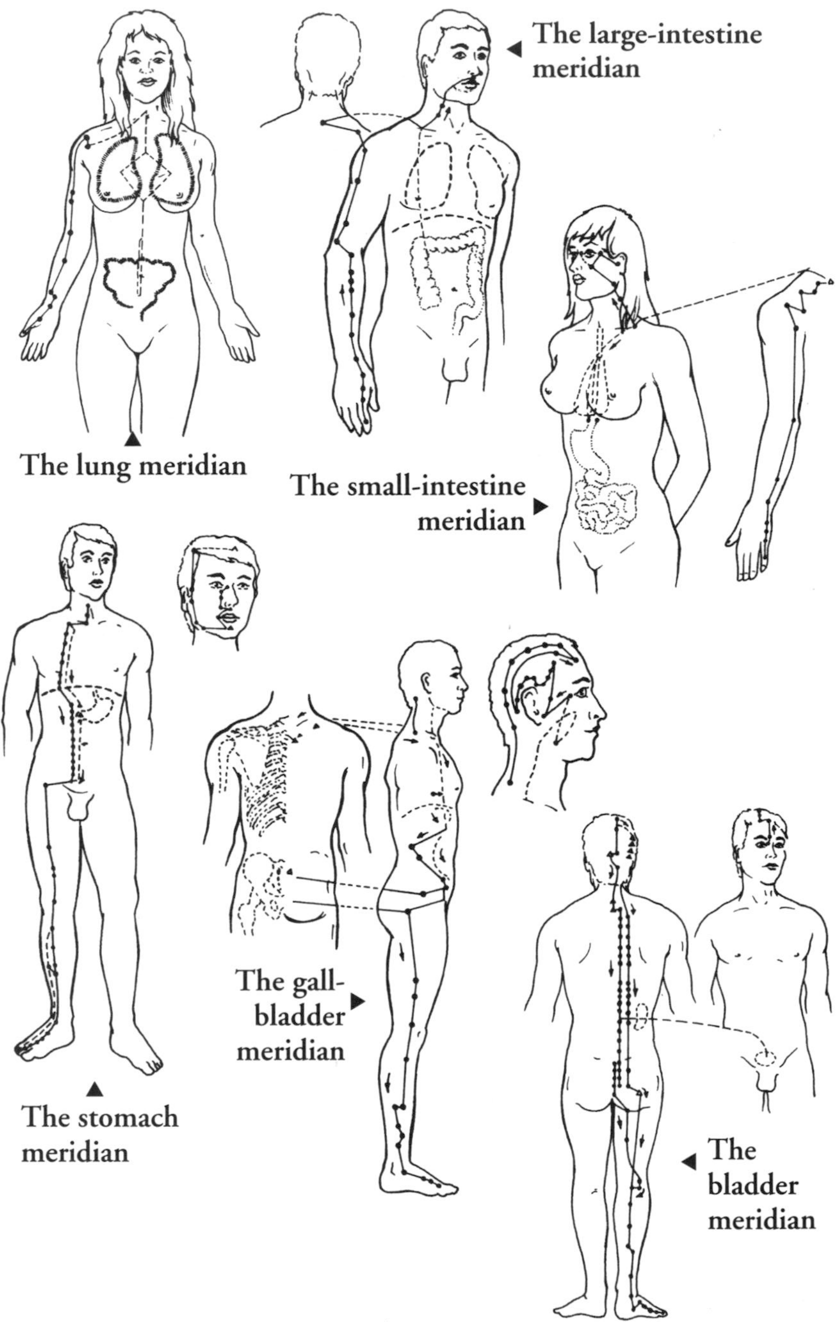
The large-intestine meridian
The lung meridian
The small-intestine meridian
The stomach meridian
The gall-bladder meridian
The bladder meridian

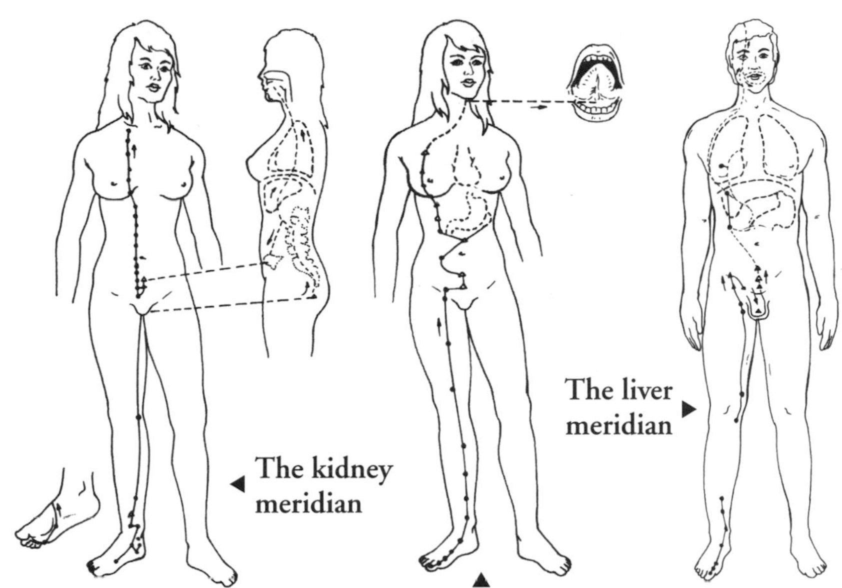

◄ The kidney meridian

The liver meridian ►

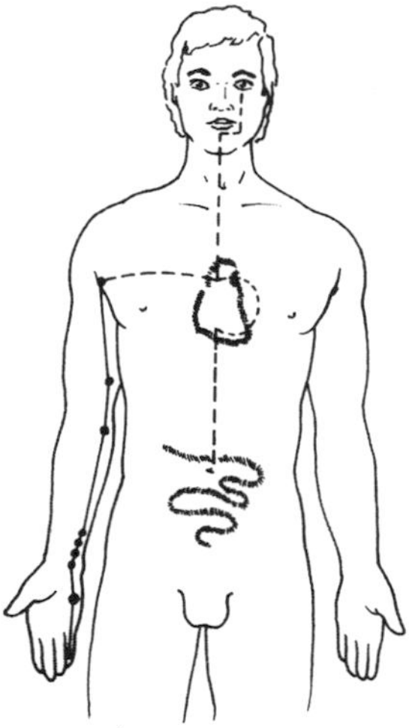

▲ The spleen-pancreas meridian

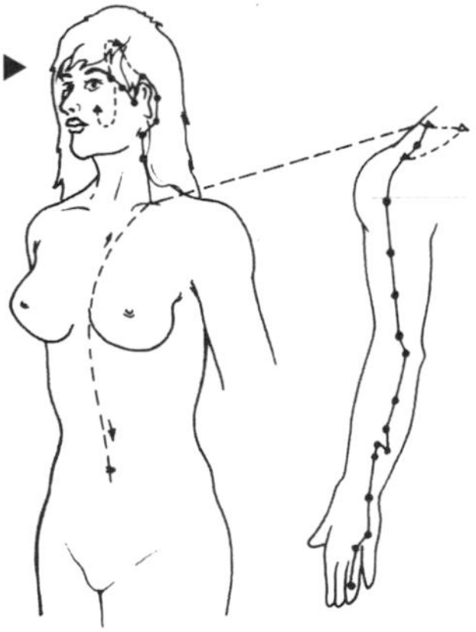

The triple-warmer meridian ►

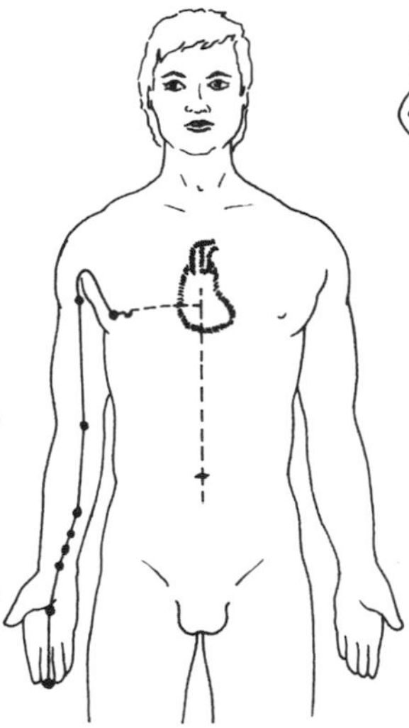

▲ The heart meridian

◄ The heart constrictor meridian

not only opposites like black and white and day and night; they are also seen as complimentary elements. They are dance partners like man and woman, like the high and low tide. Without the one, the other does not and cannot exist.

Yin and yang play together on the stage of life. They compliment each other, depend on one another, and keep each other in harmony. They come and go in waves. What goes up, must also come down again.

Yin and yang create constant movement. In life there is no stopping, no standing still, and no ending until we have drawn our final breath. And who knows if that is really the end of this mysterious existence. I suspect that consciousness always exists. It may change its shape, it may be held in this vessel for a while, but then it will reappear in another vessel.

The principle of yin and yang manifests itself in our bodies as cold (yin) and warmth (yang), ascending (yang) and descending (yin) energy, taking in substances (yin) and using these substances in physical activity (yang).

Certain body parts and inner organs correspond to yin, while others correspond to yang. The upper part of the body is principally considered to be yang and the lower part yin. The outsides of the extremities are yang and the inner sides yin.

The so-called *Fu* organs (the bladder, small intestine, large intestine, gallbladder, and stomach) are primarily yang; the so-called *Zang* organs (the liver, heart, lungs, kidneys, and spleen) are primarily yin.

A healthy body is in a state of perfect equilibrium between yin and yang. If it has become disharmonious, meaning more yin than yang or vise versa, it can be brought back into a perfect state of balance by treating it with either acupuncture, moxibustion, corrective diet, meditation, Qi Gong or Tai Chi, or a mixture.

The Five Elements

In China, it is said that everything in the universe corresponds in some way to the five elements of earth, fire, wood, metal, and water. These elements continuously interact with each other inside our body. The inner organs are matched with the following elements:

Earth—stomach, spleen, pancreas
Fire—heart, small intestine
Wood—liver, gallbladder
Metal—lungs, large intestine
Water—kidney, bladder

Each meridian corresponds to yin or yang and to one of the inner organs, as well as one of the five elements:

1 The lung meridian = yin/metal
2 The large intestine meridian = yang/metal
3 The small intestine meridian = yang/fire
4 The stomach meridian = yang/earth
5 The bladder meridian = yang/water
6 The gallbladder meridian = yang/wood
7 The kidney meridian = yin/water
8 The spleen-pancreas meridian = yin/earth
9 The liver meridian = yin/wood
10 The heart meridian = yin/fire
11 The heart constrictor meridian = yin/fire
12 The triple-warmer meridian = yang/fire

In acupuncture, moxibustion, and Shiatsu, individual points on these meridians are stimulated with either needles, heat, or pressure to restore the balance of yin and yang. In acupuncture, an excess of energy is dispersed by inserting and instantly removing a needle. Low energy is remedied by inserting a needle and leaving it in place for several minutes.

Restoring the balance of yin and yang is naturally our aim as well. A Reiki treatment can accomplish the restoration in a very gentle way. Certain acupuncture points can be lightly stimulated by simply resting our fingers or hands on them or by gently massaging or stroking points or entire meridians (see page 184 under the "Hanshin Chiryo", page 185-186 under "Hanshin Koketsu-Ho" and page 153-158 under "kenyoku").

The theory of the biorhythm inside the human or animal body is a very interesting theory worth exploring. It says that at specific times of the day or night, the healing of certain inner organs is naturally promoted because that's when the activity within the related meridians is greatest. When the meridians are treated during the "rush hour," the greatest possible result can be obtained.

CHAPTER 11

The Chakras

—by William Lee Rand—

The Chakras are a part of the subtle energy system and play an important role in health and healing. Understanding them can be helpful when giving Reiki treatments. Blocks and negative energy are sometimes lodged in the chakras and, if present, need to be released in order for healing to take place. These blocks can be detected with *Byosen scanning* (see page 162-163).

The chakras are like subtle energy transformers. They take the Ki or life force that is all around us and transform it into the various frequencies we need and bring it into our subtle energy system. They can also be thought of as points where the soul connects to the physical body. They appear to clairvoyant sight as wheels of various colors. When seen from another perspective, they appear as vortexes of energy swirling inward or outward from the various chakra points. They are shaped like the circular motion of water flowing down a drain.

There are seven basic chakras starting with the root chakra at the base of the spine and ending with the crown chakra at the top of the head. The frequency and complexity of the energy in each chakra increases in each successive chakra. The root chakra has very basic energy, and the energy of the crown chakra is very highly refined. The chakras are responsible for creating the various kinds of consciousness operating within our subtle energy systems and are also connected to the complete spectrum of human experience. Additional chakras are both above and below the root and crown chakras; minor chakras are in the hands, feet, knees, and other parts of the body.

Each of the chakras is connected to a subtle energy channel in the spine. The channel is made of three parts: the Sushumna at the core of the spine, considered to be the most important energy channel in the subtle energy system; and the Ida and Pingala that flow

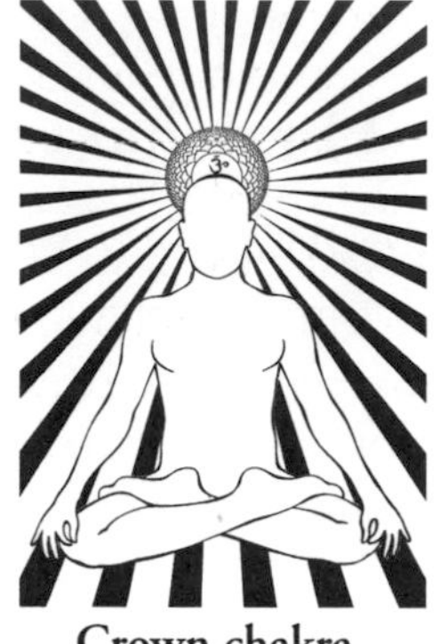

Crown chakra

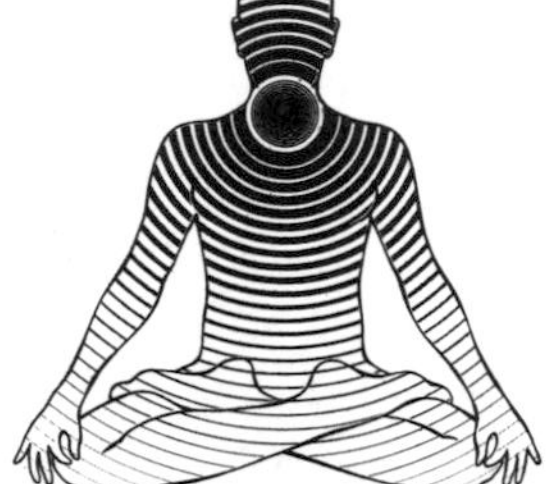

Throat chakra

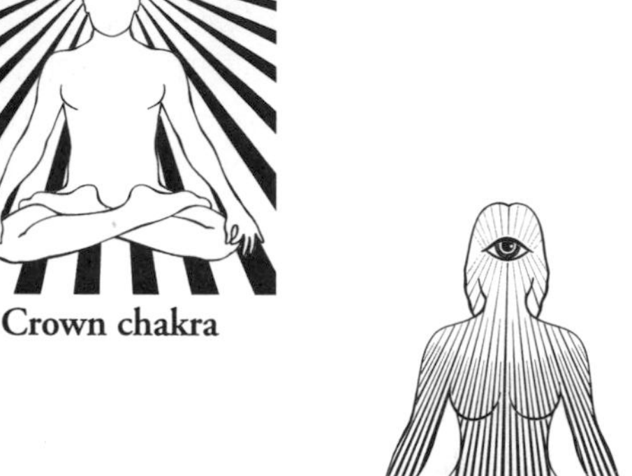

Brow chakra

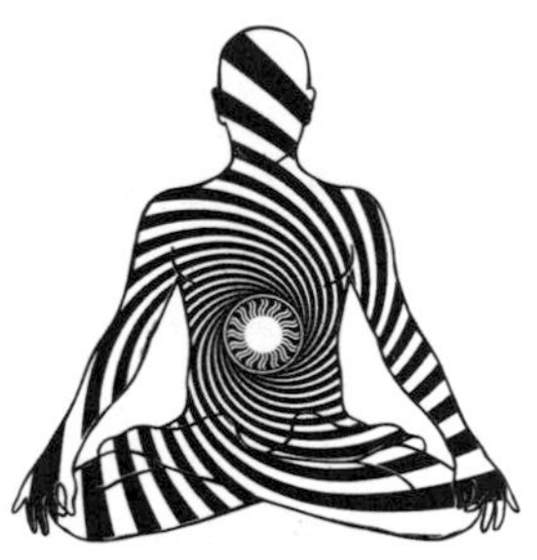

Solar plexus chakra

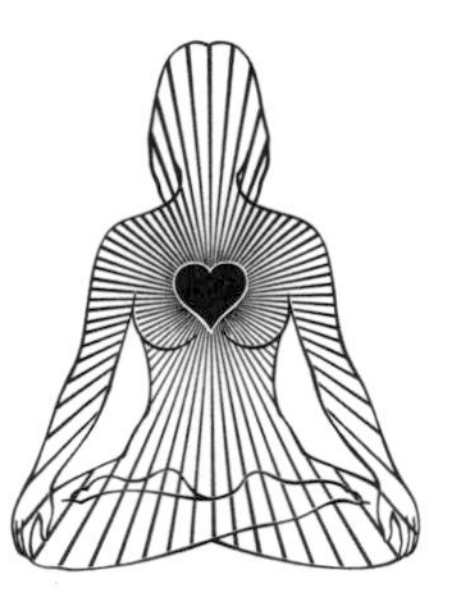

Heart chakra

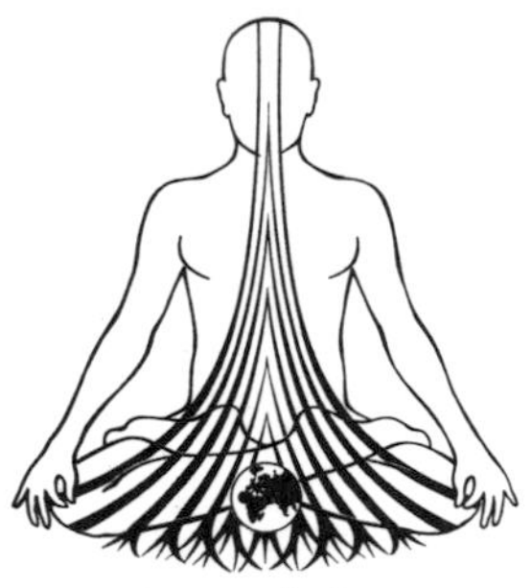

Root chakra

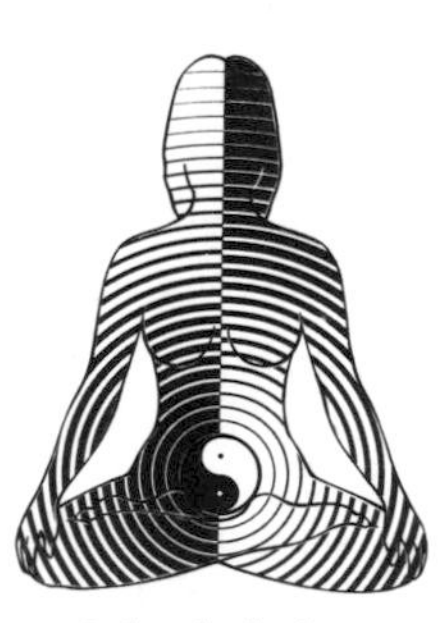

Sakral chakra

back and forth around the outside of the Sushumna. This channel distributes energy throughout the subtle energy system.

Each chakra extends out from the spine. Chakras* two through six extend both from the front and the back of the body. The front side is generally involved with receiving subtle energy and the back side is generally involved with sending energy out, although it is possible for the direction to change back and forth from time to time.

What follows is a description of each of the seven chakras.

Root Chakra

The root chakra is connected to the base of the spine and points down between the legs toward the ground. Its color is red. It connects the subtle energy system to the earth. It supports our will to live and supplies our bodies with vitality. Its energy is involved with our need for food, shelter, and the basic necessities of life.

Second or Sacral Charka

The second chakra is connected to the sacrum. Its color is orange. It is involved with reproduction, sexuality, physical enjoyment, and the attractive aspect of relationships. It is also one of the places people hide guilt and humiliation. It is the main location of the shadow self.

Third or Solar Plexus Chakra

The third chakra is connected to the solar plexus area. Its color is yellow. It brings in and sends out energy necessary for self-expression. This is also called the power center, as through it one manifests will. Confidence and purpose, as well as fear and anger, can be located here.

Fourth or Heart Chakra

The fourth chakra is connected to the center of the chest near the physical heart. Its color is green. It is related to all aspects of love and

---

* Illustrations on page 84 taken from: Sharamon S. and Baginski B. J.: "The Chakra Handbook", Lotus Light·Shangri-La, Twin Lakes, WI, 1991.

is also involved with joy, respect, and surrender. Spiritual guidance and higher consciousness can also come through the heart chakra. It is one of two important chakras through which Reiki energy enters ones system.

Fifth or Throat Chakra

The fifth charka is located at the throat area. Its color is blue. The chakra has to do with the expression of creativity through speaking and writing. It is also involved with contemplation, and some of the aspects of thinking and planning. How we relate to others and especially to groups manifests through it.

Sixth or Brow Chakra

The sixth chakra is located between the eyebrows and is also called the third eye. Its color is purple. It is involved with self-awareness, wisdom, higher consciousness, clairvoyance, simple knowing, visualization, and conceptual thinking.

Seventh or Crown Chakra

The seventh chakra is located at the top of the head and extends ways above the head. Its color is white. It connects us directly to the higher power and spiritual consciousness. It is the other important chakra through which Reiki energy enters.

CHAPTER 12

The Aura

—by William Lee Rand—

The aura is a field of subtle energy that penetrates and extends out from the physical body. It has its own consciousness, which is really your own consciousness, and it is possible to become aware of this consciousness. By meditating on your aura, you can often begin to feel or even see it. When doing this, it is possible for your consciousness to move into your aura in a similar way that you can become aware of the bottoms of your feet or the back of your neck, by simply thinking about these areas. Then you can get a real sense that who you are does not end with your skin, but extends out several feet or more into the space around you. Becoming aware of your own aura can be a beautiful and empowering experience.

Within the aura are representations of everything you have ever experienced in this life and in all past lives. Those who are highly clairvoyant can actually see the experiences in the aura of another as pictures or movies that also contain feelings and other types of awareness.

Illness first starts in the aura, often as karma brought in from past lives or as negative *Ki*, formed by your subconscious mind in this life. As time goes by, these "seeds" within the aura can become strengthened by negative energy and the experiences they attract. As this happens, these "seeds" begin to grow and extend their "roots" down into the chakras and if not healed, can eventually extend into the physical body and manifest as dysfunction and illness. Permanent healing therefore cannot stop with the physical body, or with the chakras, but must extend into the aura where the original cause resides. *Byosen scanning* (like stated on pages 162-163) can be used to detect areas in the aura needing healing in the same way it is used for the chakras and the physical body. A value of Reiki is that it works not only with the physical body, but also on all levels of our being and thus is able to bring lasting results.

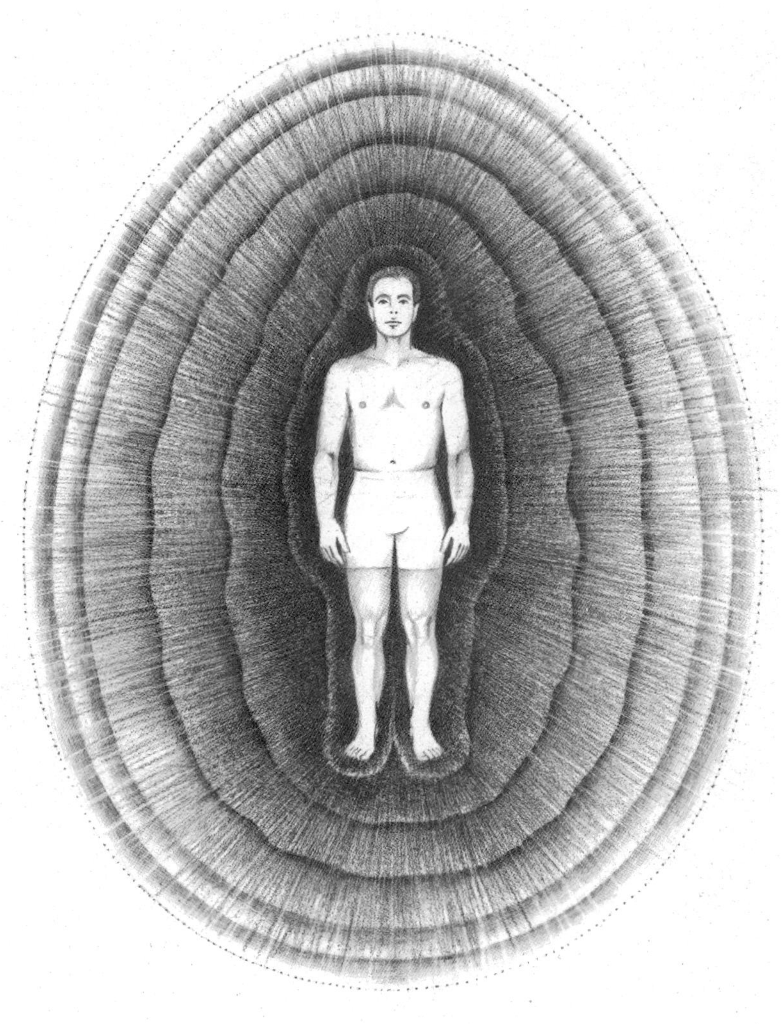

The aura* is composed of many layers or levels of vibration. The levels interpenetrate each other and are actually composed of different kinds of consciousness. Each level of the aura is connected to a respective chakra and has a similar vibration and energy as that chakra. As an example, the innermost level of the aura, which is very close to the surface of the body, is connected to the root chakra. This auric field has to do with physical health and vitality, which is similar to the energy of the root chakra. The next auric field is connected to the sacral chakra and is a little farther out. Like the sacral chakra, it has to do with physical enjoyment and attractiveness. Each successive level of the aura is connected to the next higher chakra, has a similar energy, and is a little farther from the body. The outermost or seventh level extends out about four or five feet or so for the average person.

The overall size of the aura can increase or decrease, depending on the quality of one's thoughts and feelings and on the kind of recent experiences. As an example, if one has had a bad day and is feeling tired and defeated, one's aura may recede to only two or three feet from the body. On the other hand, after receiving a Reiki treatment or an attunement, one's aura can extend out much farther than normal, sometimes as far as twenty to thirty feet or more. As you can gather, the aura not only responds to our current state of consciousness on all levels, but, in a deeper sense, actually is our state of consciousness.

Because the chakras and the aura are connected and have a similar energy and purpose, I will not further describe each of the auric levels here; you can understand the auric levels by reviewing the descriptions of the chakras.

---

* Illustration on page 88 taken from: Schneider P. and Pieroth G.K.: "LightBeings—Master Essences", Arcana Publishing, Twin Lakes, WI, 1998.

CHAPTER 13

The Journey from the Head to the Heart and from the Heart to the Belly

—by Frank Arjava Petter—

Many of us live entirely in our heads—with the exception of a few moments of romantic love. But these moments are rare and beyond our control. With romantic love we have formed an emotional attachment that binds us. Love, in this sense, means bondage. We must be released from bondage sooner or later if we want to become free.

Unconditional love is a completely different state of being, beyond the boundaries of the head and the heart. It is the ultimate flowering of the soul, a marvel occurring at the conclusion of our spiritual journey. On the journey, the first important step is to descend from the head to the heart, then ultimately move from the heart to the belly. Unconditional love only comes from the belly.

Living in the head means a calculating approach that demands rational explanations for everything, only observing with the intellect. Many modern societies place little value on living a heart-filled life. Those that have done so tended to disappear quickly. Manipulation, greed, and the desire for personal advantage seem to be much more powerful than love. But love offers a different kind of strength, the strength of openness and vulnerability. Such strength allows us to experience one of the great advantages of Reiki.

Walter has written a book with the title of *Reiki—Way of the Heart,* (Lotus Light·Shangri-La, 1996) which happens to be the exact same title I had in mind for my first Reiki book because it explains Reiki so well! After I learned about Walter's book I changed my title to Reiki Fire. Reiki is a method that brings the energy from the head to the heart. In the process of descending to the heart, a sudden explosion of emotions may overwhelm us. We may suddenly feel that we had not been living fully before we came into contact with Reiki. For the first time in our adult lives, we may feel alive and pulsating with energy. We may feel so much better than the other poor souls who are living in their heads! But here is where the trouble begins.

In my seminars I often notice that participants frown when presented with exercises emphasizing negative aspects of the psyche. Being in the heart can easily be used as an excuse not to look at these shadow aspects, which don't go away if we try to ignore them! We need to look at them, acknowledge them, and let go of them. Only then can growth occur.

In New Age circles, the qualities of the "higher" and "lower" chakras are frequently misunderstood. The higher chakras are considered to be better than the lower ones because the latter deal with "lower" energies. However, this is incorrect. In fact, the opposite holds true: The belly is the seat of our consciousness. It is our aim to find the small flame of spiritual awareness burning eternally in our hara (located three fingers below the navel). The hara is where we learn to relate to our fellow human beings without attachment, acting from spiritual emptiness instead of egoism.

Another misunderstanding is that the belly is only the seat of raw, physical power. The hara's aspect of physical power is just the starting point, the most concrete aspect of the hara. Each of our spiritual centers has many various aspects. The lowest aspect of the hara is that of sheer physical strength. The next aspect is willpower. We do not have a will of our own unless we develop our hara, which is why priority is placed upon the development of this energy center by all the forms of martial arts. However, it is also easy to get stuck in this aspect of the belly. The same also applies to many people who get stuck at the heart once they have set out on the journey to the heart. After all, the heart is such a beautiful thing. Nevertheless, it is loaded with emotional attachment, notions of how things should and should not be, and filled with moral concepts of good and bad.

Transcending the heart is a painful step. But it does not mean that we must become immoral or cold, although it may appear that way to us when the consciousness first descends to the belly. When this happened to me, I first felt sad and lonely. Emotional attachment had been the only way for me to relate to others and the world around me. The beauty of a sunset or another person's smile let overflowing emotion well up within my heart. Then suddenly, there was nothing but a feeling of emptiness in my belly. This inner emptiness extended toward others and reached them in their emptiness, in the core of their being. For a while, I did not experience any kind of pleasure. Yes, I realized later that the way I related to the outside world had simply changed. A low-burning Reiki fire had been ignited in my belly. It took me a few months to get used to it.

With the Joshin Kokyuu-Ho (see page 158 ff) breathing technique, Dr. Usui taught a very powerful way to move into the hara (Chinese: *dantien*) During the past three years, we have taught this technique to our students and have practiced it ourselves with amazing results. It appears that breathing as deeply into the belly as possible not only gives us more physical strength and Reiki energy, it also seems to fire up the immune system.

CHAPTER 14

Reiki as a Spiritual Path

—by Frank Arjava Petter—

The Usui Reiki Ryoho Gakkai claims that Dr. Usui had his satori (see chapter 1 on page 13 ff) or mystical experience about the nature of consciousness in March of 1922. They also say he conceived of the Usui *Reiki Ryoho Gakkai* in April of the same year.

The story suggests that Reiki was meant to be a spiritual path because it was born out of what we call a religious experience. Dr. Usui's aim was to impart what he had personally experienced to others. Such was the greatness and genius of Dr. Usui: the ability to channel the divine into a form that can be experienced and practiced by his fellow human beings.

In my eyes the definition of a spiritual path is a method or a technique that aids the practitioner in finding himself or herself. As many pathways to the self exist as there are people on the planet. Each one of us creates our own path as we walk it. But certain aids and techniques can make all the difference.

On your own you are likely to proceed on your spiritual journey at the speed of a bullock cart. With the help of a master, you can learn to fly and make rapid progress. With a proven system, you will advance at a steady pace.

Whether Dr. Usui was a completely enlightened master is not up to us to decide. How could we know? We can only know about our own standing. Ultimately, it does not matter because we do know he had certain insights into the deeper levels of being, which he clearly revealed to us.

In a recent conversation with Walter, he remarked that Reiki seemed to lack the *dharma* transmission in the West. As a result, it has disintegrated into what we could call a declawed tiger.

Let's put the claws back on the animal!

The Sanskrit word *dharma* means law. In Buddhist terminology, dharma means the teachings laid down by the Buddha. When followed, these teachings lead to enlightenment. Dharma has two aspects: The first is the dharma transmission—passed on from master to student. The second aspect is the realization of dharma—the student living what he or she has learned.

First of all, we need to know what the teachings are. Secondly, we need to be in contact with those who are following the teachings. Adepts who are already advanced will start to teach the beginners. Buddhism has produced twenty five hundred years of dharma transmission between Buddhist masters and their students.

Tibetan Buddhism and Zen have been particularly successful in the quest for enlightenment, resulting in large numbers of enlightened teachers. The flame leaps effortlessly from one brightly burning candle to another as yet unlit candle. Anyone who has sat in the presence of an enlightened being will know what I mean.

Unfortunately, we lack this most vital part of the path in the Reiki tradition: the enlightened souls, the elder brothers and sisters on the path who will help us along. Without their guidance, the path is very arduous.

People involved in Reiki sometimes say, "I have been guided to do this and that." However, we should be aware that what we call "guidance" may be an excuse to not take responsibility for our own actions. The fact is that each of us is solely responsible for everything we do, say, think, and feel. The skill of always acting in a totally responsible manner is an important one to take along the path. Responsibility allows us to find total freedom.

Of course, nothing is wrong with being guided. We are all familiar with the feeling of being pulled toward something like the moth to a flame, without the involvement of our will, our desires, or our ego. But it is far from the norm. We are usually the ones making the decisions, especially in terms of our financial or emotional well-being.

Whenever we doubt our own motives, we should ask ourselves whether an action done out of this motive will make us more loving and compassionate. The answer to the question will come easily. If we feel guided to follow a certain path, and the answer to the question is "no," it is important to be strong and stick with the "no." Then we are exercising our own willpower, even if it is against our own financial or emotional advantage. This dignity enables us to draw on tremendous power.

Another common phrase in Reiki circles is: "Reiki will take care of it." But, in reality, Reiki does not take care of it, whatever it may be. Either we do or we don't. Especially when our egos are involved, when we make unethical decisions that only support our advantage as an individual or group, Reiki does nothing. It doesn't stand in the way of our growth, even if our growth passes through a destructive phase. We need to take an active role in deciding what to do and what not to do. We shouldn't give our power away—not even to Reiki!

Because many of us don't have the guidance of an enlightened master, or at least the guidance of an advanced practitioner on the path, we must rely on Dr. Usui's legacy. What has he left us in terms of dharma? As far as I understand, we have the Five Reiki Principles inscribed on Dr. Usui's memorial stone, the *Usui Reiki Ryoho Hikkei* (Dr. Usui's Reiki Handbook), the Meiji Emperor's poems (see page 284 ff), *Gassho, Reiji-Ho* and *Chiryo*, as well as many other original Reiki techniques used by Dr. Usui. In addition, we have some guidance from Kimiko Koyama, the previous president of the Usui Reiki Ryoho Gakkai, which I will discuss subsequently.

The Five Reiki Principles

The more I understand the workings of energy inside and outside of myself, the more I realize that when we live the Reiki principles, they are actually all the ethical guidance we need. However, it is not the act of chanting them that creates changes but allowing them to be our guiding light. When we chant them, which is best done by learning the following Japanese words , their meaning should reverberate within our hearts.

We have been teaching the original Japanese pronunciation of the Reiki principles to hundreds of participants in our seminars. Many of them really appreciate first-hand knowledge of the spoken Japanese language. In order to learn the proper pronunciation, readers with Internet access can listen to Chetna, my wife, say them at either William Rand's homepage or our homepage.[24]

Here are the principles and their pronunciation:

Kyo dake wa (kjoh dakeh wah)—just for today
Okolu-na (ikaru-nah)—don't get angry
Shinpai suna (shin-pie sue-nah)—don't worry
Kansha shite (kansha she-the)—be grateful
Go wo hage me (gyo-o-hage me)—work hard
Hito ni shinsetsu ni (heeto knee shin-set-tzu knee)—be kind to others

The *Dr. Usui Reiki Ryoho Hikkei*

Dr. Usui and his successors gave this handbook to every Japanese Reiki student. It was later translated and published under the title *The Original Reiki Handbook of Dr. Mikao Usui* by Mikao Usui and Frank Arjava Petter.[8]

The Meiji Emperor's Poems

The intent of the Meiji Emperor's poems is similar to that of the five Reiki principles. They are meant to provide down-to-earth guidelines for an ethical existence on this planet. This type of spiritual poetry exposes us to transcendental values that can carry us beyond our small egos, beyond the limitations of our individual selves.

Read these poems on pages 284 ff very carefully. It's best to read them out loud or have your partner or friend read them to you. Savor every syllable of these poems as if they were a delicacy—this is what they are!

Gassho, Reiji-Ho, and *Chiryo*

According to Ms. Koyama, Dr. Usui said that his Reiki system was based on the five Reiki principles and what we can consider to be the three pillars of Reiki—*Gassho*, *Reiji-Ho*, and *Chiryo*. Without these components, Reiki has no wings. Over the past few years, profound changes have taken place within us and within our students. We are certain that the practice of *Gassho* Meditation, *Reiji-Ho*, and *Chiryo* (see page 146 ff) have played a very important role in these changes. Anyone who practices these techniques won't regret it.

The Five Objects of the Reiki Ryoho

According to Kimiko Koyama, the five objects of the *Reiki Ryoho* are:

1.
*Tai*体 (body)—*Ken*健 (health)

The body is the temple of God. Knowing this, we should take care of it and worship in it. Ultimately, we will not be able to endure the experience of enlightenment without a healthy body. We can make the body strong with Reiki, meditation, proper diet, and. . . laughter!

2.
*En*縁 (relation, connection, fate, love, karma)—
*Bi*美 (beauty)

Beauty and love go hand in hand. If you see the beauty in every being sentient or insentient, you are bound to live a peaceful and fulfilled life.

3.
*Kokoro*心 (heart and mind)—
*Makoto*誠 (sincerity, authenticity)

Kokoro, the unity of heart and mind, is already mentioned elsewhere. The way to achieve this unity of heart and mind is by being our authentic selves. (Arjava, the spiritual name given to me by my master Osho, means "authentic. ")

4.
*Sai*才 (talent)—*Chikara*力 (power)

Talent and power go together. When we follow our talent, the result is a power that no one can resist. There's no need to fear our own abilities!

5.
*Tsutome*務 (duty) —*Do*働 (work)

Our duty is to work on ourselves. In whatever we do, we should give the best we have. There's no need to hold back what we can give to others—and to ourselves.

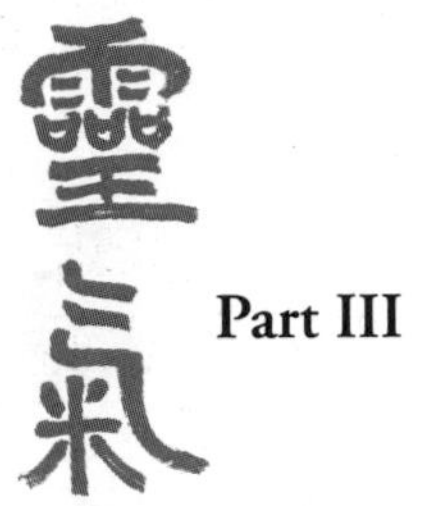

Part III

REIKI PRACTICE

世のそとはいかがあらむと
かたつぶり
をりおり家をいでて見るらむ

: 114 ***The Snail***
What is going on
Out there
That is how a snail
Comes out of its house
To take a look

CHAPTER 15

Reiki Training

—by William Lee Rand—

Reiki got off to a somewhat restrictive start when Hawayo Takata brought it to the West, but after she passed, it has gone the other way. Now people teach Reiki with complete freedom. This freedom allows for experimentation and the development of new techniques. But at the same time, the lack of any rules or guidelines has allowed some Reiki training to fall short of what people need to understand Reiki and how to practice it.

Some classes now offer all levels of Reiki, including the master level, in one day or in one weekend. Although the time frame is possible, the quality of the training leaves something to be desired. In talking to students who have had the training, I found they left the class confused and didn't really understand how to give a treatment or an attunement. Some don't even know the symbols or who Dr. Usui is. Yet, they have been given a Reiki master certificate!

Those who have taken such training without any other Reiki training or interaction with other Reiki people think the way they learned is how Reiki should be taught. Being a master and told that they can teach, they teach classes of their own that end up being even less effective. In this way, some people are getting training that really does not do Reiki justice and isn't fair to the students.

When the students find out training is supposed to last a much longer period of time and they were supposed to have practice time in class, they realize they need to take the training over from a teacher with better standards.

Although the situation is unfortunate, I look at it somewhat philosophically and reason that those who are really interested in Reiki will take the classes again from a good teacher.

Minimum Standards Needed

What standards are appropriate for Reiki training? I like to think in terms of two levels of training. The first or basic level is what has been in use to teach the majority of Reiki classes around the world. It involves about the same amount of class time that was given when Reiki was first brought to the West. The level of training is good for anyone wanting to use Reiki for oneself, family, and friends. It is also appropriate for many people wanting to start a professional practice or to teach. Remember, Reiki is very simple, and elaborate training is not necessary. Many good teachers have been produced through the basic level of training.

However, for those who plan to be a really good teacher, I suggest starting with the basic training listed below, and then practice. When ready, they can take one of the longer teacher-training programs available. What follows is an outline for the basic training for each degree.

A class manual is given for each level. Also, students should be allowed to tape record the classes and take notes.

Reiki 1

Training should take a minimum of one day, although some instructors teach it in two or two and a half days. The minimum subjects covered should include:

1. The history of Reiki.
2. What is Reiki and how it works.
3. The five Reiki principles.
4. The Reiki I attunement. Some schools can offer one or two attunements. Others can offer four..
5. Demonstration and practice time to give complete Reiki treatments to others and oneself.
6. Optionally, some of the Japanese Reiki techniques such as the Gassho meditation, Joshin Kokyuu-Ho, Reiji, Kenyoku, and Byosen Scanning.
7. Additional exercises or meditations, at the discretion of the teacher.

Reiki 2

Training should take a minimum of one day, although some instructors teach it in two or two and a half days. The minimum subjects covered should include:

1. A description of all symbols, including how to draw them, what they mean, and how to use them.
2. The students should be encouraged to memorize the symbols and a test should be given. This is important because if a student cannot remember how to draw the symbols, he or she will not be able to use them.
3. The Reiki II attunement. Usually teachers give one or two attunements.
4. Practice time in class to use the symbols so the student knows from experience what the energy of each symbol feels like.
5. Optionally, more Japanese Reiki techniques such as: Enkaku chiryo, Koki-Ho, Shu chu Reiki, and Gyoshi- Ho.
6. Additional exercises or meditations, at the discretion of the teacher.

Reiki 3A or Master Practitioner Level

Most instructors teach the class, although some teach only the complete master-teacher training. This class can be taught in one day, although some instructors may teach it in two or more days.

The minimum subjects covered should include:

1. A description of the Usui master symbol or the master symbols used in the style of Reiki being taught. I say this because systems other than the Usui system use different master symbols. Instruction should include how to draw the symbol, what it means, and how to use it.
2. The students should be encouraged to memorize the symbol and a test should be given. This is important because if a student cannot remember how to draw the symbol, he or she will not be able to use it.
3. Reiki 3A master practitioner attunement. Usually teachers give one attunement.

4. Practice time in class using the symbol for treatments so the student knows from experience what the energy feels like.
5. Additional exercises, techniques, and meditations at the teacher's discretion.

Reiki 3B or Master Teacher Level

The class can be taught in two days, although some instructors may teach it in three or more days.

The minimum subjects covered should include:

1. A talk about what it means to be a Reiki master including, the responsibilities involved.
2. Optionally, additional master symbols from other systems. If covered, steps 1 & 2 from Reiki 3A should be included.
3. The Reiki 3B master teacher attunement. Most teachers give one attunement, although some use two or more.
4. Demonstrations that carefully show how attunements for each Reiki level are given.
5. Practice time in class giving each of the attunements.
6. Discussion on what subjects to teach and time answering questions.
7. Additional exercises, techniques, and meditations, at the teacher's discretion.

Higher Level Teaching Programs

These programs are recommended for those who may have never taught a class before and need additional support in becoming a good teacher. They are also for anyone who wants to round out their teaching style, add depth to their presentation, and attain a higher level of professionalism. The programs vary from teacher to teacher, so it is important for you to check the curriculum of each program before deciding to enroll. Time for completion for one of these programs is usually between three months to a year or more. Some of the aspects the higher level training may include are:

1. Reviewing all Reiki class levels one or more times is often a requirement.
2. Co-teaching one or more of each of the classes with a certified teacher.
3. Experience doing as many as 100 or more Reiki treatments using treatment forms.
4. A written test is often a requirement.
5. Some require book reports or writing papers on various Reiki subjects.
6. Other programs are composed of much class time with the teacher and cover a wide range of subjects, including metaphysical and physical anatomy, hand positions for various conditions, personal evaluation and healing, meditation, and spiritual development.

CHAPTER 16

The Relationship Between Reiki Teacher and Student

—by Walter Lübeck—

A review of the spirit of Reiki would be very incomplete without some explanation of the complex dimension of the teacher/student relationship. This topic, which is already delicate, is particularly complicated and not always easy to understand when it comes to Reiki. So here are a few basic explanations in advance.

We have many teachers in our lifetime such as our parents, siblings, relatives, schoolteachers, trainers, friends, "coincidental" acquaintances, advisers, colleagues, seminar leaders, and authors who speak to us through books, magazine articles, films, or plays. Some of them also teach us something on the spiritual level or something that at least helps us walk our spiritual path, our path to the light and to love. We even listen to some of our teachers when they try to give us something important to take along on our path.

In addition to the informal spiritual teachers, there are also those who we more or less consciously choose as such so that they can help us on our path. Some accompany us only for a brief time, while others are with us for many years. How much a spiritual teacher can do for us depends upon his or her competence, commitment, the conditions surrounding the encounter, our will to get involved, and the stamina that we display as students.

Perhaps you have at some point asked the ticklish question of why an individual actually needs a spiritual teacher. The answer to this question consists essentially of two perceptions:

1. The eye cannot see itself—it needs a mirror for this purpose. Human beings can only recognize and learn to sincerely accept what they truly are in the mirror of another person who is clear, loving, and truthful in the respective encounter. The other person doesn't have to *constantly* be clear, loving, and truthful for this

purpose. It is absolutely adequate for this person to show these qualities during encounters that are important for the student's spiritual growth.

2. The fundamental principle of homeopathy, a method of natural healing established by the German physician and pharmacist Samuel Hahnemann, says: "like cures like." (Latin: "Similia similibus curantur!"). Applied to human emotional life, this means that the injuries, frustrations, and fears we have suffered in relationships can only be healed in symbolically similar relationships. The individual imprisoned within himself or herself can be redeemed and become aware of the light within through the encounter with another person who, in critical situations similar to those that have caused the blocks, is willing to allow the divine to work through his or her being. Please note: *One person* does not redeem the other!

Time and again, I meet individuals who think the theme of the teacher/student relationship is certainly important—but only for other people. These individuals think that they have personal direct conversations with the creative force and everything necessary takes place in this way. I do not doubt that there are people who can attune themselves to the divine in a direct manner. However, it seems audacious to me when people trapped in their fears, blockages, and frustrations believe that they can trust in their own very great ability to resonate, which is ultimately the foundation of every form of communication with the realms of light. With absolute certainty, the creative force will listen to each prayer, take our concerns seriously, and answer appropriately from the spiritual perspective. However, without training and help, working on ourselves, and a true expansion of consciousness, are we all capable of hearing the answers "from above," recognizing the divine advice, accepting it despite the turbulence of everyday life and putting it into practice in an appropriate manner? And whether we perceive and accept the divine counsel is the decisive point if we want to shape our lives in a more spiritual manner through divine help.

Reiki as a Spiritual Path

In addition to its significance as a holistic method of healing, the Usui System of Natural Healing is a spiritual path for anyone who uses it accordingly. By becoming involved with the universal life energy in theory and practice, we can reconcile with our divine center in terms of our consciousness and increasingly allow its loving light to radiate out into the world. To support this process, we need Reiki treatments on a regular basis (no matter which degree), a basic openness for the transformation of the life structures, and an awake consciousness that pays attention to *what* is set in motion and *how* it moves. This is a serious motivation for learning to love life, ourselves, and others, as well as assuming responsibility for our personal matters and supplementing the qualities necessary for taking the spiritual path of Reiki.

However, in order to work with Reiki in the first place, most people require an initiation and basic training in how to treat the universal life energy. This is where an encounter with a spiritual teacher occurs, possibly for the first time. But this teacher does not have to be a spiritual teacher in the narrower sense. In contrast to other spiritual paths, it's enough for the Reiki Master to correctly gain mastery in his or her craft, which means being capable of giving initiations that work and teaching the students the fundamental treatment techniques. So the Reiki path has a very simple beginning. This fact has played a major role in how quickly Reiki has spread throughout the world.

The Reiki path can function as a spiritual path in several different ways.

1. You can repeatedly treat yourself and others with Reiki. When doing so, always be sure to truly be *in* the situation and not let your consciousness disappear from the here and now. Think about the life principles and try to integrate them a bit better into your life with each passing day. Make an effort to develop more love, personal responsibility, and consciousness. This type of path includes many monologues, writing a diary, conversations with other Reiki friends, and the ability to motivate yourself time and again in your progress. At some point, spiritual experiences will

manifest themselves in your life and you will probably recognize some of them for what they are. Their meaning may somehow become perfectly clear to you.

2. You continue your Reiki training and complete the 2nd Degree. The symbols and mantras are part of this level, including some techniques of how to use them. The type and number of these that are taught depends upon the Master teaching them. However, power intensification and distance and mental healing will probably be explained to you. Now you can follow your Reiki path and discover who you are with more tools, but basically in the same way as explained under 1.
3. You complete the Master Degree and learn to initiate others into the Reiki system, imparting the respective basic knowledge to them. In principle, you can also take this step without the necessity of a spiritual teacher. It's enough to be trained by someone who can effectively initiate you and convey the appropriate knowledge to you. The Master Degree has the variations of just letting yourself be initiated and otherwise continuing to work with the possibilities of the 1st and 2nd Degrees, as well as meditating with the Master symbol and its mantra. The initiation into the 3rd Degree helps many people to open up more to Reiki and progress more easily on their path as a result. This development is not a certainty since it depends greatly upon the external circumstances and the personal background precondition of everyone involved.

   If you decide instead to train others, in time you can have spiritual experiences through the initiations and technical instructions that you give, whereby the information under 1. still basically applies here.
4. You open up to a spiritual teacher/student relationship and participate on a regular basis in the training activities of the degree that you have learned. You may take private lessons and also come to terms with your teacher and his or her instructions, in addition to your involvement in Reiki. In my experience, this path is the most effective. However, it is not simple or comfortable.

No matter what basic path you decide upon, if you seriously apply yourself to it, Reiki will lead you to experiences that can help you to perceive the light within yourself. Its healing rays will open up more and more doors within your being. Like other spiritual paths, Reiki consists of techniques and know-how, as well as meaningfully applying these to human relationships. If you do not take the techniques and knowledge seriously at the beginning, Reiki cannot help you very much. However, if you still take the techniques and knowledge very seriously at a later stage, it is quite possible that you will also block your progress.

Here is a story on this topic: Many years ago, I learned Tai Chi Chuan. I exerted a great deal of effort to move exactly like my master, and I progressed with time. At some point, I no longer perceived any differences in my movements and those of my teacher. He apparently had the same opinion since he did not improve anything on my form for a number of practice hours. Then, one day he suddenly said to me: "You are doing the form wrong!" I was quite astonished! "Why? " I responded, "I'm doing the positions exactly like you are!" "Exactly," said my master and smiled at me.

When you do not learn a form, you have no ladder to reach the next highest level. If you do not set the form aside as soon as you master it, you will eternally tie yourself to the ladder instead of entering and exploring the higher levels. Spiritual paths often appear to be made of paradoxes.

The Spiritual Relationship Between Reiki Teacher and Student

A Reiki teacher can initiate you and show you the applications so that you can gain a variety of practical uses from your new abilities with their help. Yet, the path is the goal!

How do you apply your knowledge and abilities? Do you really pay attention to the new qualities that increasingly enter your life through Reiki or do you ignore parts or all of it? Do you only apply certain Reiki techniques instead of drawing on the abundance? Why do you prefer certain techniques and avoid the others? It's possible that the neglected tools in particular are what you need to progress at all—or even progress especially well! Do you believe that you are progressing on your path? Which criteria do you use to evaluate your progress? Are your values suitable for this purpose? Or have you just accepted them from your—possibly unresolved—past for these purposes, without knowing if they are actually unuseful for a spiritual approach to life?

Do you orient yourself on your feelings, which ultimately are just based on patterns of reactions to stimuli that you learned as a child and teenager, in order to stabilize a specific behavior or a certain personality structure? Or are you willing to consider yourself and your feelings as two different entities and accordingly understand that you produce your feelings? When you want to produce this energy in certain qualities, can you also let it be created within you in other strengths and characteristics? Do you want to learn how to do this? Do you want to assume responsibility for what you bring into this world? Or would you prefer that others continue to bear the blame?

It isn't simple to deal with these questions, especially not alone. It helps to have a spiritual teacher who will try to help you answer these and other difficult questions and approach yourself and your life in a new, more constructive way. However, this is not the actual spiritual path—but an important foundation for it. A human being does not become more spiritual by gathering knowledge, even though properly applied knowledge can offer good support on the path to the light. The spiritual path does not consist of accumulating power, even though the acceptance and loving approach to the personal opportunities for power can enormously promote spiritual growth in certain situations. The spiritual path is not for workaholics, even though it is frequently very important to work on ourselves until we drop.

Even just finding the proper proportions is not easy. And the higher we climb, the more difficult and dangerous the whole thing becomes. If we want to find our way in a totally foreign land, we are well-advised to hire a trustworthy guide who is familiar with the conditions there. Precisely this—nothing more and nothing less—is the role of a spiritual teacher. Setting ourselves in motion, selecting the approximate direction, and moving in it—these are things we must do ourselves.

Is a Reiki Master Automatically a Spiritual Teacher?

As already discussed above, a Reiki Master is not necessarily a spiritual teacher. And he or she doesn't have to be one. The minimum requirements for a Reiki Master are the ability and know-how for initiating others and training them in the fundamental application of the universal life energy. Incidentally, other traditions also have similar situations. Chinese qi gong and Indian yoga have certain schools that officially differentiate between "technique teachers" and "path teachers. " I don't think there's anything wrong with this. In Asian martial arts it is also completely normal to subdivide the Master Degree into several different titles in order to appropriately describe the varying qualifications. Every person can learn something—always! Why not stand up for what I can do—and for whatever is still my learning task. This is also love, clarity, and truth!

Reiki Masters can become spiritual teachers if they continue to work on their personal development. However, this does not always occur automatically. A Reiki Master who has only been active for a short while may teach in a very spiritual manner, while someone who has held seminars and Reiki sessions for many, many years may still have a very limited understanding of the spiritual dimension of the Usui System of Natural Healing.

What exactly can happen in a spiritual teacher/student relationship? Without more closely illuminating this topic, it is difficult to translate the above explanations into practical terms.

How You Can Recognize a Spiritual Relationship Between Teacher and Student

First, I would like to explain the meaning of a few words that are frequently used in this context so that we have a mutual point of reference.

The term "spiritual" is derived from the Latin spiritus—spirit. So it means "related to the soul or the divine." "Esoteric" is also a word borrowed from Latin. It means "related to what is concealed." The opposite of this is "exoteric": related to what is apparent."

A few examples may make the meanings easier to understand: When a businessman buys new equipment for his company in order to better produce his products, this is a materially oriented action. But this does not mean that it is compulsive or objectionable in a moral or ethical sense. If he *also* considers environmental protection, better working conditions for his employees, an increased quality of his products, and a new way of designing his personal work situation that promotes his own development as a human being and corresponds with his own nature, then this entrepreneur is acting in a spiritual way.

Even if he doesn't read any relevant books or attend seminars, let alone know the "jargon." If he uses oracle work, numerology, channeled messages and rituals in order to find the optimal machines for him and his business at the best price and transform the resistance of his personnel against uncomfortable innovations into constructive activities with new possibilities, then he is acting in an esoteric manner. An esoteric action is not necessarily always ethically correct, meaning that it is not always simultaneously spiritual. Many people primarily get involved with the wide-ranging interesting field of esotericism in order to gain advantages over others who are less informed and/or trained. And this may just be to always get the free parking space when they *want* it, having the good-paying new job promised to them ahead of all the other applicants, passing an exam, being respected, and winning at Lotto.

In summary, this means that:

- Materially oriented people first think of their own well-being and survival, as well as (possibly) the concerns of those closest to them (family, circle of friends, etc.).
- Esoterically oriented people use knowledge about the laws of nature, of which many people are quite ignorant, and the resulting abilities in order to master the challenges of their lives.
- Spiritually oriented people *strive to the best of their knowledge and good conscience* to take care of themselves and those closest to them *in the way that is most individually appropriate to him*, as well as providing *opportunities* for as many other people/beings for individual personal development and lasting improvement of their quality of life.

The definition of the term "spiritual teacher" can be derived from this description. Within the field that they teach, which is Reiki in this case, such instructors attempt to contribute not only to their own well-being but also to human and material welfare, as well as the individual character development of the students entrusted to them, as well as they can in their own personal way.

Everything human is fundamentally finite and therefore imperfect. Demanding perfection in any form from a human being shows a deep lack of insight into human nature, which has apparently been designed this way by the creative force. We inhabitants of the earth can strive to the best of our knowledge and conscience when it comes to fulfilling our private and professional obligations—but we will always somehow fail or produce inadequate results. If we are spiritually oriented, we will constantly attempt to learn as much as possible from our errors and do what is best for the whole of Creation. We will be willing to question those convictions that we considered to be truths yesterday when we become aware of other viewpoints that are better suited for our individual growth, happiness, and well-being.

Once we are Reiki Masters, our students will learn many useful techniques and information from us; however, when training others we will repeatedly mention that perhaps tomorrow there will be even better techniques. Our students' attitudes toward what they have learned and how they use it will be very important to us. Promoting human development whenever possible will become increasingly more important than imparting practical contents because we have understood that it is dangerous for everyone involved when immature people have a great instrument of power placed in their hands.

As spiritual teachers, we will challenge our students to seriously question our convictions and viewpoints so that they will become independent and develop a responsible way of thinking. Not only will we oppose blind faith on the part of our students but also vehemently question it when our students display it. Time and again, we will point out that there is something to be learned during every phase of life and that it is very valuable to occasionally "drink from other sources"—to study with other teachers who are competent as human beings and in their field of work. In the case of doubt, we will risk the harmonious relationship with our students if we are pressured to impart certain teachings that we feel are not ethically correct or for which our students are not mature enough at this time. This also applies if we believe that other things are more urgent for our students to work on in order to achieve lasting happiness, well-being, and success. This last point in particular naturally requires some personal stability on the part of the teacher and the ability to show integrity in dealing with our own fears in relation to not being loved and acknowledged, as well as the securing of our own material survival and well-being.

Consequently, a spiritual teacher's deep love is not necessary shown by smiling all day long, always being nice and friendly, and speaking with a gentle voice. Instead, we are strong enough to openly show a variety of feelings to every person and assume responsibility for these feelings. Instead of saying: "It's your fault that things are going so poorly for me," we can say something like: "I'm sad and angry. I'm not ready to deal with this situation right now." Our love is expressed in that we help our students develop themselves and allow personal responsibility, love, and consciousness to grow, even against our own personal interests in case of doubt.

However, despite all of the provocation and resolution that a spiritual teacher may display, we always ultimately leave it up to our students to decide what to do, what to become involved in, and how and when they will approach a task.

This point also includes the idea that a spiritual teacher is only permitted to clear the stones from the path of a student when they objectively represent a serious danger to the student's progress *and cannot be removed by the student.* If this principle is not observed, the spiritual and specialized competence of a student can never develop. This situation will also create an unhealthy dependence on the teacher.

Students naturally profit the most from longer periods of training, whatever form these may take. In this way, maturation in terms of both the professional and the human aspect will occur in a more lasting manner. The deeper the human relationship and the trust that grows between the teacher and student in many mutual experiences, the more essential contents can be imparted and the more extensive the transformation can be. Yet, a spiritual training relationship must also include a phase of cutting the umbilical cord after a certain period of time. In the ideal case, both parties should handle this process in a correct and loving way. This last section of the apprenticeship time should then lead into a friendly and essentially egalitarian human relationship. In my opinion, a spiritual apprenticeship with a teacher should not last much longer than two years, but definitely no longer than five. Shorter periods of time simply do not allow enough depth to be achieved. Longer periods of training lead all too easily to dependencies. However, there are naturally exceptions—especially when dealing with spiritual topics.

The end of a period of spiritual training naturally does not mean that there is nothing more to be learned from the teacher. However, after the umbilical cord has been cut, this should occur on a basis of equality between two human beings in something like project groups.

A Few Thoughts in Closing

Spiritually oriented teachers do not deal with ultimate truths and solutions to problems that always function. Instead, they seek honest human encounters, as well as information and skills that can be used in a practical manner, which they impart to others and constantly continue to develop.

- Spiritually oriented teachers have not arrived at the goal but have walked the path to meaning and love longer and more attentively than their students.
- Spiritual teachers do not advertise with the lowest prices and fashionable trends but with who they are and the message they have to offer. Even the best teachers cannot be effective if they do not open up to their students.
- The length of the teacher/student relationship depends on the extent of the student's desire to advance.
- Spiritual teachers do not always have to be understanding, but they should impart understanding.
- A serious student has serious doubts about the path and the teacher.
- Spiritual teachers do not have the essential task of giving answers, but of asking questions. Spiritual teachers don't misuse the students' situation economically or sexually and don't make them become dependent on them.

CHAPTER 17

The Reiki Symbols and Mantras

—by Walter Lübeck—

There are many stories and mysteries related to the symbols and mantras*. of the Usui System of Natural Healing. People often believe that just the knowledge of the symbols and mantras will open the door to Reiki, making the initiations superfluous. Why this is not true will be explained later in greater detail. This chapter discusses the meaning and application of the symbols and mantras of the 2nd and 3rd Reiki Degrees. To begin with, here is a general overview of the topic.

Symbols and Mantras in the Various Spiritual Traditions

Symbols and mantras are used in almost all of the spiritual traditions for meditation, personal development, healing, and energy work. They can basically be divided into two types: such that can create ***subjective changes*** and such that can create ***objective changes.***

Symbols and mantras that can create subjective changes:
Modern examples of this are affirmations and the conscious use of symbolically significant objects (the cross, yin/yang symbol, circle, stop sign) or forms and colors in order to produce certain moods and associations. In the esoteric context, these types of symbols are used particularly in Chinese feng shui—the art and science of designing working and residential spaces, as well as gardens, in a way that supports life and healing.

We can use any sign or picture, any word, and practically any object in this way, as long as we have certain strong emotional asso-

* The "symbols" refer to the three signs of the 2nd Degree and the one sign of the 3rd Degree. With their help, Reiki can be used for many purposes in a very simple way. The "mantras" are the words associated with the symbols. They activate the symbols.

ciations—such as those based on our education, cultural background, membership in a religion, or impressive personal experiences—connected with it. The effects achieved in this manner vary greatly and are not the same for everyone, especially not unprepared users, since the personal, emotional valuation of what is perceived determines the type, length, and intensity of the effect.

Symbols and mantras that can create *objective* changes:
Examples of these are the Reiki symbols and mantras, as well as runes, magical amulets, and the holy mantras from the Indian Vastu, the "Mother of Feng Shui." With the help of the latter, the energetic qualities and living atmosphere of rooms can be changed.

In order to deal with these tools, we fundamentally require instruction from someone who has already used them within a certain objective framework and has the ability of transferring the system of his or her energy work. If we want to do it on our own we have to soulfully attune ourselves to the respective system. This naturally also includes the correct use of the symbol. One example of learning this correct use can be seen in Tantric Buddhism, the spiritual path from which Reiki was originally born. Here, precise rituals and the recitation of the initiation mantra—often more than 100,000 times during favorable astrological periods—is connected with a sequence of visualizations of mantras and invocations of the respective deities in states of deep meditation. Mikao Usui used these possibilities, which were probably shown to him by his abbot friend at a Zen monastery in Kyoto or by monks in the Mount Kurama Monastery, during his 21-day retreat on Mount Kurama. This mountain, a place of power close to the Japanese city of Kyoto, has been famous for centuries.

If we use the first, less complicated and strenuous path of passing on this knowledge from person to person—instead of the complex procedure of the second path—this can be called initiation. In accordance with the characteristics of the respective tradition, this path can be translated into practical terms in a wide variety of ways. Examples of these are: Reiki initiations, Taoist initiations (Qi Gong and magic), transmissions of Barraka by the Sufis, Shaktipat in Hinduism, Tantric initiations, Kriya Yoga, shamanic initiations into a certain medicine power, initiations into a magical lodge in a certain degree of power of a deity.

Basically, symbols of the first category that are thematically suitable and not too general can be turned into tools with defined functions in the scope of the second category through the appropriate exercises and a great deal of personal commitment (devotion), as well as the spiritual support of beings such as angels. In order to do this, it is usually necessary for the respective person to have been in a state of enlightenment for a time or can consciously enter into it. The function of a mantra or a symbol is not clear and distinct before it is transformed into the second category. The same sign, word, or sentence can be associated with various functions, deities, and energies in the different esoteric traditions. It may be quite powerful in one case, but have a very gentle effect in the next.

Dr. Usui had to attain access to a lost tradition and took the above-described path when facing the problem that the symbols and mantras he had found in the Sanskrit writings had no effect on him. Through his three-week meditation and fasting on Mount Kurama, he connected with the spiritual traditions behind the writings, the symbols, and the mantras. In this way, he achieved the ability of being a Reiki channel, initiating others into this spiritual tradition, and shaping and using the tools of this heritage.

So the symbols and mantras are not Reiki. Instead, it is only possible to use them through the traditional initiation within the scope of the Reiki system. Otherwise, they are signs and words like any other and are sometimes used in completely different contexts in the everyday language of Japan: for example, temples and gravesites are decorated with them. In such cases, their meaning is not directly connected with the purposes familiar from the Reiki practice.

When the symbols and their mantras are imparted correctly within the scope of the Reiki initiations, we can rely on their power and the effects. Symbols and mantras that have been looked up in books or learned from friends without the personal initiation are simply characters outside of the esoteric context—but not precise, powerful tools of energy work.

Additional Symbols and Mantras

Time and again, new symbols and mantras that the respective Reiki schools have considered part of Reiki have emerged in recent years. Here are some thoughts on this practice:

The traditional Japanese Reiki system was divided into a number of degrees. The sixth degree, called Shoden, was the lowest (today we call it the First Degree in the West). In turn, this was divided into *Loku-To* (6th Degree), *Go-To* (5th Degree), *Yon-To* (4th Degree), and *San-To* (3rd Degree). Initiations and instructions in relation to the use of the Reiki symbol of the 2nd Degree (according to the Western system) did not take place at this training level. Among other things, its contents were: contact treatment, development of subtle perception, and spiritual instruction, as well as the techniques described in *Reiki—The Legacy of Dr. Usui* by Frank Arjava Petter. Consequently, these degrees basically correspond with the 1st Degree of the currently applied Western classification system.

The next highest degree is *Okuden*, which is separated into two sections: *Okuden-Zenki* (first half) and *Okuden-Koki* (second half). The symbols were taught in the first section. Students learned about distance healing and mental healing in the second section. In addition, the Reiki Masters taught the methods discussed by Dr. Usui in the Questions and Answers section of the above book by Frank Arjava Petter. This degree basically corresponds with the 2nd Degree of the classification system generally used in the West today.

The following degree was called *Shinpiden*. The Reiki teachers selected very few students to learn this degree. Once students were initiated into Shinpiden, it was possible for them to receive the permission to professionally treat others.

Only students who had completed Shinpiden could become assistants to the teacher. This position was called *Shihan-Kaku*, which means something like "teaching assistant. " When the teacher thought it was appropriate, he or she would give respective students the permission to hold their own meetings and have their own students. This position was called *Shihan*, which means "teacher. " However, this term also includes a feeling of authority, exemplariness, strength, and wisdom.

This degree basically corresponds with the 3rd Degree (Master/ Teacher) of the classification system generally used in the West today. In the Japanese system, the symbols were the same as those that we have today in the 2nd and 3rd degree (of the Western system).

Dr. Usui did not teach any other degrees and symbols. If additional tools of this type are included in Reiki instruction, this can occur in two different ways:

1. The symbols and mantras that belong to another form of energy work—meaning that they function with other energies—are used. In this case, the simple term of "traditional Reiki" is erroneous because these systems do not work with Dr. Usui's System of Natural Healing. Rules other than those of Usui Reiki are in effect here.

2. Additional symbols and mantras are included in the power flow of the Reiki system in the same way as Dr. Usui made the traditional four symbols and mantras into a part of the Reiki tradition that he established. This is naturally possible since Dr. Usui was a human being and any of us can achieve what he accomplished, at least in principle. However, this is not a simple task. It requires the permission of the patron deity of Reiki, Dainichi Nyorei, who will be discussed in detail later. At least as long as it is necessary for the respective person to enter—consciously or unconsciously—into a state of enlightenment for a time, it is necessary for us to have the appropriate expertise about the tasks to be accomplished.

Just as the traditional four symbols and mantras intensify Reiki, and/ or let it be manifested more intensely on the level of material reality, or direct the flow of the universal life energy directly into certain vibrational levels or areas of a living being's energy system, additional symbols and mantras can have a similar effect. For example, there are four of these types of tools in *Rainbow Reiki* for bringing the universal life energy directly into the areas of a being's energy system that are connected with the elements of earth, water, fire, and air. However, these additional aids should naturally not be called "traditional Reiki according to Dr. Usui."

Why Is It Advantageous to Learn More About the Reiki Symbols and Mantras?

It is very important for Reiki friends to explore the symbols and their mantras. The better we understand what they mean and where their roots lie, the easier and more precisely our intuition will function. This also makes it easier to adapt the energy work with Reiki to the respective circumstances and thereby more strongly develop our creativity in solving the problems that may possibly arise. In addition, a deeper understanding of the symbols and mantras helps us use the Usui System of Natural Healing as a spiritual path and shape it in a way that is appropriate to our own personal nature. We could say that the symbols and mantras are the key to the palace gates.

The Best Way to Approach the Reiki Symbols and Mantras

Respect—Not Pretense of Piety

The symbols and mantras of the 2nd Degree are tools that can be used with the appropriate initiation within the scope of the Reiki system. The inner child—the body consciousness that is responsible for all of the practical directly applicable esoteric abilities, the true emotions, and the memory—judges the importance of a matter with which someone is involved according to the attentiveness and love that is practiced in the process, as well as the respect shown it. So when we treat the tools of the 2nd Degree with mindfulness, love, and respect, our inner child knows that these are important things, pays more attention to them, and reacts accordingly. Furthermore, it can more easily grasp the traditional essence of the symbols and mantras, to which the rational mind has very little access, through this type of approach. In no case should the symbols and mantras become meaningless fetishes or holy (sanctimonious) relics. We absolutely should not worship them, and it isn't advisable to always "look holy" when they are discussed.

Examples of the correct approach to the "tool box" of traditional Reiki include drawing the symbols and mantras with complete mindfulness and not tearing, bending, or throwing away the paper used for practicing them. Instead, this should be burned in a special ritual and stored beforehand as flat paper or rolled up and bound. In the same way, a sign drawn improperly during practice should not be crossed out or improved. Instead, simply start over and be careful to carry out the process of making the symbol more correctly this time. The purpose of practicing and using the symbol is not to create something that looks right, but correctly carrying out the process of creating the symbol and repeating the mantra.

Private—Not Secret

Since anyone can visit the 2nd Degree seminar—and the tools of the Usui System of Natural Healing can now be found on the Internet, as well as published in the form of books and magazine articles, the symbols and mantras certainly can't be called secret. However, I think that it is still appropriate to keep them private because of spiritual reasons—this means not "decorating" postcards, business cards, t-shirts, buttons, homepages, posters, house walls, or ashtrays with them. At most, they would have a subjective effect in these places since this type of use is not Reiki energy work. The more clearly they are reserved for a certain distinct area of functions and tasks, and the more we treat them with respect, the better our inner child will understand what the symbols and mantras means. Consequently, it can use them more effectively within the scope of conscious energy work with Reiki.

Developing a Personal Relationship with the Symbols and Mantras

When we approach **the symbols and mantras with the right attitude of consciousness**, we will quickly develop a personal relationship with them. Then we can increasingly perceive and experience their qualities. In addition to the technical knowledge about their function and position within the Reiki system, this consciousness work is an important key to the essential spiritual significance of these tools. In any application, they will not only fulfill their function but also evoke their associated spirits to the person using Reiki. This will increase the vibration of this individual's being and improve his or her intuition. So the signs teach in a way that is scarcely comprehended by the rational mind, yet definitely can be verified through the respective person's experience in terms of effective personal growth.

The Meaning of the Reiki Symbols and Mantras

The following section is intended to support a better understanding of the various functions and the position of the symbols and mantras in the Reiki system. It is important to deal with them in a clear manner that is free of superstition. This is the only way that they will develop their full effects in the long term, allowing us to work with them in a creative manner. To better differentiate them, the abbreviations of the symbols and their mantras with which most initiates are familiar will be used here.

This basically applies: Draw the symbols with the initiated hand* or mentally. Then recite the related mantra three times quietly or mentally.

According to how the initiation into the Second Degree has been performed, it is possible to either use the other Reiki symbols individually or only together with the CR (power intensification) symbol. In case of doubt, ask the Reiki Master who performed the initiation whether he or she always transmits the Second Degree symbols together with the CR during initiation or initiates all of the symbols individually. When the CR is used together with the other symbols during all of the techniques, this ensures proper functioning in any case. The CR, with the exception of some applictions within the Master degree, is almost always used *after* the other symbols. The "materializing" CR intensifies the effect of all Reiki symbols. Therefore, it should be always used to intensify the effects of the respective Reiki energy work.

The description of the symbols here will primarily include their applications and information important for the personal Reiki path. Their historical and mythological background will only be touched upon since this topic is too extensive for the scope of this book.

---

* This is generally the hand that is more skilled mechanically and better developed in the kinesthetic sense.

The Transpersonal Contact Symbol HS

Function: Together with the CR, the HS serves to connect us with the levels of light of the high self. Every human being has three archetypal partial personalities: The inner child, which is the body consciousness responsible for genuine and vital feelings, the memory except for short-term memory, our vital energy, and our will to live, as well as all of the practical spiritual abilities (extrasensory perception, the ability to act on the level of energy) and contact with the high self. The inner child "thinks" in chains of associations, momentary feelings, symbols, and patterns, the high self watches over the life path of the respective individual; it can mostly be found outside of time and space in the light worlds of the subtle beings. It maintains contact with the Akasha Chronicles. The middle self is the everyday consciousness. It evaluates the information of the five "conventional" senses (seeing, hearing, feeling, smelling, and tasting), organizes the habits (routine behavior in each area), and practical/logical thinking. Most people experience the middle self as their ego.

Time and space are not the inevitable constants from the material level here. On the high level of the self, the circumstances are organized according to stronger or weaker resonance in relation to the spiritual, procedural linking of the senses between beings and other structures of existence. So if there is a high degree of similarity between the nature of two beings, how they have their experiences in life, and/or the essential theme of their experiences, they will be close as long as their experience processes possess these qualities. Distances, past, present, and future are not an issue here. This makes it possible to do distance treatments and establish mental contact with other beings, spirits (such as angels, gods, power animals, and elves), and places of power. Contact with more than one recipient or delayed perception and Reiki transmission also becomes possible as a result. This connection between the beings is reciprocal, which means that information and true spiritual forces also flow back and forth in addition to the Reiki.

Interpreting the meaning:

a. "I am making contact on the level of the high self." or
b. "The Buddha within me connects with the Buddha within you."

c. The HS also symbolically represents the Buddha consciousness, the ability of enlightened beings to extend their mind beyond the boundaries of personal structure and time and space. The Buddha consciousness includes everything and identifies with nothing. Within it, the ego is transformed to the true divine will that supports the life process in all of its decisions without any reservations. Because of this quality of the HS, the transference of any hostile forces—destructive in the spiritual sense—is impossible. The Buddha consciousness has no room for evil. However, spiritual energies and information can move back and forth through it. So the HS serves, for example, as one of the essential tools of Rainbow Reiki for the creation of Reiki essences and astral distance perception, as well as establishing contact with spirits and the light worlds in general.

The HS symbol is a Japanese-Chinese character that is listed in its individual components (syllables) in any relevant dictionary. However, holy symbols also have numerous levels of meaning in countries other than Japan. Consequently, special Buddhist works, which were available at university libraries with Japanology departments, had to be consulted for some of the translation work.

Meaning for the personal spiritual path of Reiki practitioners: Individuals who have been initiated into this symbol and its mantra and use it on a regular basis with mindfulness, respect, and commitment will experience a progressive expansion of consciousness and increasing possibilities for transforming the ego. This development can be accelerated and intensified through special Reiki techniques.

The HS should be always used together with the CR in order to work effectively.

Some Reiki techniques for which the HS is required: distance treatment, cleansing the energy of a room, a Reiki shower, power-place work, subtle communication, Reiki channeling, astral journeys, creation of Reiki essences, journeys through time, clearing karma, and contacts with the high self and the inner child.

The Symbol of Freedom SHK

Function: Normally, the SHK is mainly used for mental treatment, which means the dissolution of disharmonious thought patterns (inappropriate habits) in the unconscious and subconscious areas of the middle self. In addition, it serves as a spiritual protective sign by dissolving the shadow on the mental level that means unconscious, disharmonious behavior routines. This reduces the importance of confronting the themes of the shadow in the outside world. For example, when used on a regular and correct basis, this sign can make it possible to more easily and constructively master the feared astrological transits of the "hard" planets Saturn, Uranus, Neptune, and Pluto. The consistent use of mental healing also supports our conscious orientation in the "here and now." This not only supports the flexibility with which we approach the various situations and experiences of life and our vitality, but also our spiritual development to a considerable extent.

In order to explain this effect on our spiritual development, we need to take a look at the developmental history of a human being: Behavioral routines are formed immediately after conception on the basis of our outer experiences and their use within the framework of our innate constitutional possibilities. During the so-called non-language phase—which is the period of pregnancy and the first year of life up to the development of the ability to speak—the types of behavior that are formed generally condition us more intensively than any other period of life. This type of imprinting is very difficult to change. If at all, we can only talk about or reflect on it in a symbolic manner since the consciousness was not yet organized by language at the time of its creation. This type of behavior is related to everything that we can regulate without our consciousness—for example, the bodily functions of standing, walking, jumping, dancing, talking, reaching for something, facial expressions, gestures, how we speak, inflections of our voice, and automatic emotional reactions*, "spon-

* So-called *secondary feelings* that are differentiated from the spontaneous *primary feelings* of the inner child, which cannot be reproduced through similar forms of stimulation.

taneous judgments," being afraid of something that may or may not objectively correspond to the intensity of the fear in terms of the actual threat it represents, shame, guilt feelings, disgust, self-doubt, inferiority complexes, and the like.

Every time that we subjectively have an experience that is particularly meaningful and makes a strong impression upon us, or when we have a similar experience repeatedly within a short time span, habitual patterns are being imprinted on us. Certain behavior routines can't simply be adapted to the needs of the present by the built-in updating program within human nature. These forms of behavior are usually shaped during childhood in order to adapt us to our family surroundings. So-called "guard programs" attempt to maintain these patterns that were previously necessary for survival and use all of the forces of the subconscious mind that they can reach for this purpose. So fear or aversion is created during contact with certain situations, information, or people capable of changing this behavior pattern: we miss the train, lose the keys to the car, provoke accidents, get a headache or stomach ache, or fall into a trance that obscures consciousness in order to direct our attention from the surrounding world to some inner process, secondary feeling, daydream, or memory.

In short: All behavior automatisms that are not adapted to the present needs of a human being so that they promote and stabilize happiness, success, health, and well-being prevent us from living a good life and keep us tied to the past. In addition, these types of habits also impede the flow of the genuine emotional energies of the inner child. Happiness and love, success and relaxation only exist in the here and now. The so-called spiritual awakening, the experience of light, is also only possible when we have learned to be completely in the here and now and be completely present within our true selves. If it is used correctly and on a regular basis over a longer period of time, the mental healing technique is extremely useful in order to achieve this goal.

This is why I call the SHK the "symbol of enlightenment."

Interpretation of the meaning: SHK means "habit" or "disposition/tendency toward..." Within the scope of the Reiki system, it can only be used together with the CR. The symbol that was the forerunner for the development of the SHK can be seen at almost any Japanese cemetery. It is connected with the Bodhisattva Avalokiteshvara (Sanskrit). This deity is synonymous with Kannon, a goddess who is revered as *Kuan Yin* in China and *Tara* in Tibet. She stands for all-embracing love and omnipresent compassion. In most parts of Asia, Avalokiteshvara is the symbol of redemption from the bonds of the material world. However, this process is not conceivable without enlightenment.

The SHK symbol was developed from a sign of the Indian spiritual language of Sanskrit. This approach was customary through some centuries in Japan. Many holy symbols were created that people still work with in Shingon, being influenced by Esoteric Buddhism.

An additional esoteric meaning is protection from the loss of spiritual consciousness through attachment to the material world. In this respect, SHK is also a symbol of spiritual cleansing from attachments. Within the Buddhist context, this probably also relates to the Amitabha Buddha (Japanese *Amida).* The Bodhisattva Avalokiteshvara is a manifestation of Buddha Amitabha.

Meaning for the personal path of Reiki practitioners: In addition to the usual effects of the individual techniques, correct work with the SHK symbol develops our understanding of the present and our true, divine selves. We increasingly learn to be with ourselves and in the present. The qualities of spiritual love grow, and we can experience the opening of our hearts.

Some Reiki techniques for which the SHK is required: mental healing with and without affirmations, creation of Reiki essences, Reiki amulets, and chakra healing.

Please note: The SHK is not a protective sign in the sense that it will protect your car against accidents, theft, or even a traffic jam; it won't stop bad people from entering a house or make it unnecessary to watch small children. It becomes a protective sign when we work with it, creating lively and effective habits in the process.

Mental healing does not hypnotize us or influence us in any other way with respect to our happiness in life. The sole function of mental healing is to guide Reiki directly to the energetic vibrational level of the habitual patterns. Once there, it can cause a human being's own self-repair and updating programs to increase and improve their activities. When affirmations are used within the scope of mental healing, they focus exclusively on the effect of Reiki on the area of habitual patterns thematically connected with their message.

The Power Intensification Symbol CR

Function: The CR is mainly used in the Usui System of Natural Healing to intensify the Reiki force and the respective effects of the symbols. One more important characteristic of the CR is that it can focus Reiki on a specific place in space, practically concentrating it. Through the (counterclockwise) direction in which the symbol is drawn, an intensification of the material effects can already be recognized. If it were to be constructed in the other direction, it would be more abstract and less effective in guiding Reiki into the material level. The CR can be also used several times, if required. In this case, the Reiki force would flow even more strongly when the recipient has basically already accepted it. So the fundamental rule that Reiki is absorbed by the body consciousness can't be invalidated with this sign.

In Japanese Shinto magic, the CR symbol also serves as an aid in turning wishes into reality (among other things).

Interpretation of the meaning: The actual meaning of CR is: "Reiki should now flow (more intensely) in this place!"

CR can be literally translated as the "Emperor's decree" or "The Tenno's Instructions." Here is an additional esoteric meaning: "Realization of the Buddha nature," which represents the spiritual awakening within the material body.

The CR symbol is an ideogram—a pictorial depiction of a specific idea. In this respect, we can only interpret the symbol—and not, like its mantra, look it up in a Japanese dictionary.

Meaning for the personal spiritual path of Reiki practitioners: Through correct use of the CR, the effects outlined above—and others—can be produced within the scope of practical energy work. CR can be a great help in allowing us to increasingly grasp the spiritual nature, the divine essence of every material object and every being, on an intuitive level. Instead of orienting our everyday behavior patterns toward the illusion of the material hull, we live according to this new perspective. In addition, CR points out the fact that every concrete manifestation, every experience is always proceeded by the intellectual concept, the idea, the mental structure. In this respect, the CR expresses the well-known truth that each of us decides to which thoughts we will give our attention and therefore determine the quality of the things that we encounter in the outside world.

Some Reiki techniques for which the CR is required: The CR can be employed together with any Reiki technique for the intensification of the effect. Furthermore, it serves to focus Reiki in terms of location.

Please note: In order to precisely focus Reiki in terms of location, be sure to correctly place the CR symbols required for this purpose. The CR symbol should always be drawn *in a counterclockwise* direction when viewed from the perspective of the energy source. It is a law of nature that subtle energies are accelerated through a field that turns counterclockwise and are drawn to the other side of this field on the material level with intensified effectiveness. (This rule does not relate to the direction of rotation in whirls.) It therefore applies equally north or south of the Equator.

The Master Symbol DKM

Function: The DKM reveals the Buddha nature within the scope of Dr. Usui's Reiki system through the initiations. This occurs to the point that the universal life energy can be extensively directed from the divine light worlds into the material level of existence. However, in order to make this possible, the symbols CR and HS are also required. On its own, the DKM is too abstract to accomplish a sustained practical effect.

Interpretation of the meaning: The DKM represents the Buddha consciousness. It is closely connected with the main deity of Shingon, *Dainichi Nyorei*, who is known in China, India, and other Asian countries as Buddha Vairochana (Sanskrit term for "He Who Is Like the Sun.") Since the end of the 1st Millennium, he has been equated with the sun goddess Amaterasu, the main Shinto deity. An analogous translation of the DKM, a Japanese-Chinese character, is "great enlightenment." An important part of the symbol means "great light." The connection also becomes obvious here. Buddha Vairochana is one of the five transcendent Buddhas. Of these five, the highest—the Original Buddha—is said to be in a state of perpetual meditation. The *mudra* (Holy, symbolic hand position) of the highest wisdom or of teaching is associated with him. Other symbols attributed to him are: the sun and the wheel of the teaching (Dharma Chakra). In Shingon (literal translation: School of the True Word.) the Japanese variation of esoteric Buddhism, Vairochana is the Sun Buddha. He is the center of the spiritual void and the highest mandala of Shingon. The four so-called Dhyani Budhhas* revolve around him like planets around the sun. Buddha Vairochana gives the human being striving for spiritual awakening the holy powers of the Three Secrets of the body, speech, and mind as an aid for the great venture. Only a person initiated into these powers can comprehend the absolute truth, which Vairochana represents. The Sun Buddha unites within himself a completely harmonious relationship of the six Buddhist elements of earth, water, fire, air, space, and consciousness.

Meaning for the personal spiritual path of Reiki practitioners: In my experience, the most effective use of the Master Symbol is to initiate people into the various Reiki Degrees with it. Initiating others and teaching the Usui System of Natural Healing is the path of the Reiki Master for achieving perfection. Through deep immersion in the enormous spiritual power field of the holy symbols that are activated in the initiation and the resulting awakening of the Reiki powers in the initiate, the initiating Master experiences a significant increase of his or her own vibrations. Connected with the spiritual consciousness work and other Reiki methods, enlightenment and an entire series of extraordinary spiritual powers *(Siddhis)* can develop over time. However, this does not require initiation into the Master Degree since every Reiki initiate is connected with the DKM, even if it is only actively used by Reiki Masters. An acceleration of spiritual awakening is basically possible in any of the degrees.

---

* All five transcendent Buddhas are basically one and the same being, which in turn represents the entire Creation. However, for the purpose of teaching meditation, the five Dhyani Buddhas are differentiated. The highest of these is Vairocha. The others are: Amitabha, Amoghasiddhi, Akshobhya, and Ratnasambhava.

Some Reiki techniques for which the DKM is required: Initiation rituals in the 1st, 2nd, and 3rd Degrees, as well as initiation into the genuine special symbols that guide Reiki directly to certain areas of the energy system, such as the chakras or the areas of the four energetic elements; symbol meditations and special forms of the Reiki shower.

Please note: The Master Symbol DKM is not a "super intensification symbol." The CR symbol is available for strengthening the flow of Reiki and intensifying its effects. Dr. Usui assigned each of the four Reiki symbols a task that is clear, distinct, and different from that of the other symbols.

An Error: The Master Symbol Does not Describe the Quality of Reiki

It has become common to use the Master Symbol instead of the Reiki Symbol because some people believe that it is the essence of Reiki. But this is not true. Incidentally, the Master Symbol is basically just a simple character that can be found in any good Japanese dictionary. No one will experience true spiritual development or become healthy just by looking at this sign. We can do energy work with this symbol only when we have been initiated into its use in the sense of the Usui System of Natural Healing and employ it correctly. If this were not the case, every student of Sinology, every Chinese and Japanese would very quickly achieve the best of health, holiness, and Reiki abilities.

Basic Information about the Use of the Symbols and Mantras

The symbols and the mantras that are used in the Usui System of Reiki are not effective in themselves. They only achieve their power in relation to Reiki through a person: a) who has been initiated into the symbols and mantras in a direct spiritual line; b) who uses the symbol with its respective mantra; and c) who properly uses the traditional basic method. If one of these conditions has not been fulfilled, it is very likely that the Reiki effect will not occur.

It is absolutely necessary to learn the symbols and mantras by heart—they cannot help us if they are filed away in a notebook.

When speaking of them without intending to use them, always use the abbreviations.

It is important to learn, understand, and use the signs and mantras correctly. This will support personal development with Reiki.

For the purposes of energy work with Reiki, the symbols do not have to be drawn or written by hand. They are ultimately activated through a precise mental image and the powers of the mind. Yet, whenever possible, correctly draw the symbols in the air with the initiated hand (for an application) and say the mantras aloud in order to practice. By hearing them and the kinesthetic sense, they will be increasingly anchored within you. In the course of time, they can help your Reiki practice become easier and more effective.

The mechanically more skilled arm is initiated because the kinesthetic sense within it is more fully developed—so it is better to practice with it. However, Reiki is naturally in the entire body! This is why the other hand and the feet do not need to be initiated. The initiation of other body parts does not have a positive influence on an individual's personality or health. However, if you use the 2nd Degree methods it will have a positive influence on your health and spiritual development. The benefit of an initiation results from the practical application of the abilities it has awakened.

If you try to always use the processes, symbols, and mantras in a correct way, new programs or habitual patterns that you can confidently fall back on will result in time. Then Reiki can be set into motion solely on the basis of the strong wish to help. But this requires a long period of attentive practice for most of the students.

Try to increasingly understand and comprehend the symbols and mantras with both your mind *and* your instinct. The Usui System of Natural Healing will then offer you more opportunities than you can take advantage of during one lifetime.

Please note: The feeling of energy produced when forming the sign does not mean that it can be used for power intensification. You are just feeling the vibration showing that it is now activated and you can work with it.

Is Reiki Just Something for Buddhists?

This impression could easily arise because there has been so much information about Buddhism in this chapter. Yet, there is only one creative force. This force and its messengers has been given different names in the various cultures and regions of the earth. The heart of each spiritual path—if it does justice to its name—is basically the same. We do not have to become Buddhists to learn or practice Reiki. Members of any faith can learn Reiki without leaving their own spiritual tradition. Reiki offers us a personal encounter with the divine—independent of any church, sect, or holy writing! *Reiki is.*

CHAPTER 18

The Japanese Reiki Techniques

—by Frank Arjava Petter—

This chapter explains the simple but very effective Japanese Reiki techniques that did not make the journey from the East to the West. With the exception of one, all the techniques were taught by Dr. Usui. We learned some from Mr. Ogawa and some from other Japanese Reiki teachers, whereas other techniques were found in three original Japanese manuscripts given to us by Mr. Ogawa about one year before his death.

Why Hawayo Takata and those who came after her did not teach these techniques remains a mystery to me because we know for a fact that she learned and practiced them herself. In fact some of the techniques—especially a breathing technique called *Joshin Kokyuu-Ho* and the intuitive, pretreatment prayer/technique called *Reiji-Ho*—are the basis of what Dr. Usui taught. In Hawayo Takata's diary, she wrote that she was taught these techniques in May of 1936. Some of the early Reiki masters initiated by Hawayo Takata were given a booklet that her daughter had printed, and the booklet is an additional resource to prove the authenticity of the techniques.

The Reiki techniques we use in the West are neither wrong nor inferior to those practiced in Japan. They are simply different. The Japanese techniques make a wonderful addition to your Reiki toolbox. With these techniques Reiki regains its Japanese flavor.

Needless to say, Western Reiki includes many additional techniques unknown to Japanese Reiki practitioners. These Western Reiki techniques could greatly benefit the Japanese practitioners as well. If we all join hands and work together, a great deal more could be accomplished. Instead of just working for our own enjoyment and ego gratification, we have been given the ability to become a tool for the divine—a hollow bamboo through which existence can play its song. Reiki is thus an easy path. We can learn from each other, completing and expanding the work that Dr. Usui started 80 years ago.

After all, each and every one of us has received his legacy. Let's make him proud of us.

Before we begin with the techniques, here is some information on the cultural background of Dr. Usui's Japan and the Reiki system, as well as how he taught it.

Traditionally, Reiki has been and is still seen as a way of life in Japan. Selecting a Reiki teacher means choosing her or him for life. Some students may have taken 20 years to learn what we call the Second Reiki degree, while others may have never learned it. After students initially met Dr. Usui, they were evaluated in relation to their skill. The grading was done like this: The lowest degree, called *Shoden*, was divided into Roku-To (Six), Go-To (Five), Yon-To (Four), and San-To (Three). The next degree, called *Okuden*, was divided into Okuden-Zenki (first half) and Okuden-Koki (second half).

Then came the next degree, called *Shinpiden*, which was followed by Shihan-Kaku and Shihan. The teacher decided who would be allowed to take the next degree and when. Very few would be chosen by their teachers to learn the highest degree. Anyone who wanted to open a new branch of the school first needed to recruit five members.

Of course, just because the Japanese traditionally used the foregoing method does not mean we should incorporate it in the West. Our culture is very different from the traditional Japanese. The times have also changed. Life has become much faster than it was in the 1920s. In order to survive, it is important for us to go with the flow of things. Reiki is like a living being, constantly changing and evolving, growing and expanding. Every culture where it is taught brings a little extra spice to Reiki.

For many years my wife Chetna had wondered why the Reiki system we had learned in Germany and brought with us to Japan seemed very logical and somehow Western. It had supposedly been conceived by Dr. Usui in Kyoto. Years before we learned about the Japanese roots of Reiki, Chetna said that Reiki must have been created by a Western mind. We thought Dr. Usui might have been one of the rare Japanese people who think in a linear, logical manner. After eight years in Japan, during which time I had met and taught English to hundreds of people, I only met one Japanese individual who appeared to think like a Westerner. The intuitive way of thinking is neither inferior nor superior, just different from the Western approach. In my opinion the way that the Japanese think is absolutely wonderful. It will be discussed in more detail subsequently.

Since we were not able not find any solid historical evidence about Dr. Usui during the first year of our research, we started to doubt that he had even existed. Then, one day we had the great pleasure of finding Dr. Usui's grave. With the help of our friend Shizuko Akimoto, we were later able to connect with members of the Usui Reiki Ryoho Gakkai.

The rest of the story is history . . .

In Japan people tend to be quite intuitive and shy away from rigid structures, rules, and regulations. They operate mostly from the right brain hemisphere, the intuitive side. The Japanese tend to think in pictures, following their hearts and bellies rather than their rational minds. Unlike English or German, the Japanese language does not allow for absolutely precise statements. Their language orientation applies to personal communication, as well as descriptions of the healing arts.

An obvious exception to the intuitive orientation is Japanese politics, which is ruled by Confucian thought. Every little detail is planned in advance, decided and established from now to eternity. In the Japanese political system, little or no room exists for change. When an unforeseen situation occurs, the entire system simply freezes. The effects can be seen in the reaction of Japanese politicians after the terrible Hanshin Earthquake that killed five thousand citizens in 1996: Because no earthquake was expected to hit the Kobe area, the authorities did not know what to do. As a result, they did virtually nothing for several days!

Let's consider the most obvious defining factor for a culture: its language. Japanese characters—*kanji*—are pictures. Western letters are concepts, causing Westerners to think conceptually. The Japanese think in a different manner, which is more abstract than logical. As a Westerner, the conclusions drawn by my Japanese students often leave me with a giant question mark inside my head. It is by no means a negative statement about the Japanese. I love Japan, the Japanese people, and am even married to a Japanese woman with all my heart! However, I experienced plenty of confusion during the first few years of our marriage because of the cultural difference. So I would like to use the knowledge of Japan I have gained to help other Westerners understand the origins of Dr. Usui's Reiki system.

Basic Rules of the Japanese Society

Cultures evolve in a great variety of ways and are influenced by many factors, such as their geology, social systems, language, climate, and so forth. For example, one culture may have a completely opposite perception of morality, friendship, time, and space than another culture. When confronted with each other, members of both cultures will naturally feel their approach is the right one. We constantly see this happening in the area of international trade. One of my Reiki friends is married to a top manager for a large American corporation. She recently told me that after two years in Japan, he still does not understand the cultural rules. My response was that although I have been in Japan for eight years, I am still baffled time and again by the way people react to situations.

In the following section, I share my experience of the basic rules that make Japanese society tick. My experience should make it possible for you to see why such a huge gap separates Japanese and Western Reiki groups.

1. Group consciousness: the *uchi* concept of the in-group
2. Strict hierarchy: up and down relationships
3. *Kokoro*: unity of heart and mind
4. Silence

1. Group Consciousness: the *Uchi* Concept of the In-Group

I have often joked that Japanese people don't have an individual ego. But there is some truth to this! A Japanese proverb says: "The nail that sticks out will get hammered in!" The in-group has many different manifestations. The basic in-group is the family. When talking about a person's home, it could be referred to as *uchi*. The word could be translated as "my/our house," "myself," "my/our family," "my/our company," or "my/our group." The family unit has strict boundaries, excluding anyone not part of the family. The boundaries are so extreme that people don't even have parties in their homes in Japan.

The next in-group for children would be their kindergarten, school, tennis club, or university. For adults, it would be the immediate neighborhood, the company they work for, their village or city, state, and ultimately their country. The individual members will do anything for these in-groups. Within the group, Japanese people can feel safe and secure. They usually draw strength and the will to live from the group.

In terms of its geography, Japan is separated from the rest of the world. Consequently, Japanese people generally lack the sense of having neighbors or borders. When I ask my English students—who mostly come from well-educated middle to upper class families—about their neighboring countries, they seriously respond, "We have no neighbors, there is only water."

The Japanese have a very powerful collective group ego. Any Westerner who has ever been to Japan or done business here is aware of the phenomenon. Obviously, many implications come from the lack of a strong personal ego in Japan:

- People do not take individual initiative.
- People don't apologize for stepping on someone else's foot in a crowd. (Who would apologize for having stepped on their own foot?)
- People do not say "no" to each other because that would hurt the other individual's feeling. (Who would want to hurt a member of their in-group, even if that person is a stranger?)

It is incredibly beautiful to see the harmonious way in which Japanese people work together. Instead of doing their own thing, everyone is geared toward the same goal and the success of the group. The American anthropologist Edward T. Hall[25] divides cultures into *high-context* cultures and *low-context* cultures. He states that *high-context* cultures do not need to speak much because each member of the group knows the other's thoughts and feelings. *Low-context* cultures need a great deal of meetings, discussion, and posing of questions. Japan is a high-context culture, as contrasted to a low-context culture like Germany or America.

For many years, I wondered why the truth about Japanese Reiki history had remained hidden for us in the West for so long. But the concept of *uchi* gives a very clear answer. As foreigners, we do not and will never belong to the Japanese in-group. Even though I was the first person in Japan to openly teach all levels of Western Reiki, I still have not been accepted into the group of people who learned from me because I basically do not exist for them!

In theory the Usui *Reiki Ryoho Gakkai* is open to the public, but the fact is that it is a very tight secret society with about five-hundred members in Japan. One can only become a member if introduced by someone who already is a member, and if there is a space. But since the members usually stay with the group for the rest of their life, it is difficult to get in. I know of only one person, Mr. H. Doi, who has managed to become a member of the group. Through him Walter, William, and I asked the *Gakkai* in the winter of 1999 if they would be willing to have some kind of exchange with us. Mr. Doi doubted that anything would come of it, and so far we have not heard a word concerning establishing a relationship.

If you consider that the *Usui Reiki Ryoho Gakkai* has been operating since 1922 and that Japan has 120 million inhabitants, the *Usui Reiki Ryoho Gakkai* is a very small group indeed.

2. Strict Hierarchy: Up and down Relationships

There seem to be no relationships of equality in Japanese society, which is a society traditionally based on martial rules and regulations. Relationships are with someone who is either higher or lower in rank. When two or more Japanese people initially meet, the hierarchy is established within a few seconds. In the business world, when people exchange business cards, they read the card and immediately know whether the other person has a higher or lower status. If the second person's status is higher, the first person will bow more deeply. If it is lower, the first person will bow less deeply.

When people are equal from the perspective of social status, an artificial hierarchy is created. For example, when two workers of equal standing work for a company, one of them will have entered the company before the other, will have graduated from the university before the other, and will have been born before the other. The elder of the two is then called *Senpai* and the younger *Kohai*. A teacher, anyone who imparts knowledge of any kind to another person, is called *Sensei*. The boss is called *Shacho* and the manager, depending on rank, is *Butcho*, *Katcho*, or *Kakaricho*. The positive aspect of the custom is that relationships are always clearly defined and elders are given the respect due to them. In the world of Reiki, it explains why a teacher is chosen for life.

3. *Kokoro:* Unity of Heart and Mind

The concept here has already been described in detail in my second book, *Reiki—The Legacy of Dr. Usui*. To summarize: The Japanese do not divide themselves into heart and mind like most Westerners do. The word *kokoro* means a unity of both.

4. Silence

An old proverb states that "talk is silver and silence is gold." In Japan, the proverb would be rephrased as "Whoever talks is stupid!" The main focus of Japanese culture is on intuiting, sensing what the others are thinking and feeling rather than discussing it. People are meant to pick up nonverbal cues from each other so they don't have to ask personal questions that would embarrass either others and/or themselves. Just a glance out of the corner of his eyes will be enough for a master of nonverbal communication to understand whether his business partner will agree or disagree on the proposed deal and how to proceed with the negotiations. A quick glance across the room is all that is needed for something that would take a Westerner fifteen minutes to explain. What an experience it is to be part of a Japanese corporate decision-making process—no one talks, and everyone, with the exception of the foreigner, knows what is going on!

In a Japanese Reiki session, little need exists for verbal communication. Ideally, the practitioner should discover what the other person needs by using the *reiji-ho* and *byosen* techniques described subsequently.

The Development of Reiki in Japan

Quite recently, in the fall of 1997, we found out that the original Reiki system created by Dr. Usui was partially based on intuition. The practitioner was taught to follow his/her hands in the manner described as follows. Because of the many, many years invested in learning and practicing Reiki in Japan, a rigid system of hand positions and a specific amount of time allotted to treating with each of them was unnecessary. The system of twelve, fourteen, or more hand positions was created in the West. It is obvious in the chapter containing Chujiro Hayashi's Reiki manual (see chapter 19 on page 190 ff) that he did not create the "Western" hand positions. He may have developed them after he teamed up with Hawayo Takata.

Our research suggests that the Western Reiki system as we know it was created mainly by Hawayo Takata, who, despite her physical appearance, was an American. (You should not necessarily stop using the Western hand positions. They serve their purpose and are very helpful to the beginner in particular.)

Under the leadership of Dr. Usui, four meetings a month were held at the *Usui Reiki Ryoho Gakkai's* headquarters. The meetings included the activities described as follows.

The Meiji Emperor's poems were read aloud. Dr. Usui was supposedly very fond of the Meiji Emperor (see the drawing on page 285) and spoke of him with great respect. Traditionally, Japanese emperors (*Tennô*) are regarded as incarnations of a Shinto god. Even to this day, many Japanese citizens deeply revere their emperor and the entire imperial family. Photographs of the imperial family can be found in many homes of the elderly.

In political terms, the Meiji period (1868-1912) was an era of great change and unrest, a time in which many old patterns were broken and new ones were just emerging. The era must have been similar to what we are now experiencing at the beginning of the new millennium. In the early years of the Meiji period, Buddhism and Christianity were violently persecuted. When Buddhism was introduced to Japan in the fifth century, it had mingled with the original Japanese religion of Shintoism and many Japanese became followers of both faiths. The Meiji restoration aimed at separating the two religions again and turning Shintoism into the state religion. During this process, many Buddhist monks were killed, monasteries were closed or destroyed, and their inhabitants were given the choice whether to convert to Shintoism or suffer serious consequences. Many Christian groups went underground or disappeared all together.

The violence against religious groups must have been one of the reasons Dr. Usui incorporated the Meiji Emperor's principles into his Reiki work. He must have wanted to avoid the fate shared by many other energy-healing groups in his time. *Taireidou* (the hand-healing group), for example, was banned and separated into many small groups in order to survive. Dr. Usui's position before studying Reiki as the secretary to Shinpei Goto, a high-ranking politician of the day, must have also played a part in his political overtones.

I am sure his political connections and the fact that many Reiki practitioners of Dr. Usui's day were of high society (according to a 1929 newspaper article, the president of the Bank of Tokyo was a Reiki practitioner.) saved the Reiki movement from persecution. During the Second World War, however, some Reiki practitioners were worried that their group would be associated with the peace movement. Mr. Ogawa told us that for this reason the Gakkai cut down their organized activities during the war. But then they started them up again after 1945.

At Dr. Usui's Reiki meetings, attendants read the poems out loud and listened to a lecture delivered by Dr. Usui. Apparently, he was very funny and had a great deal of vital energy. Many people would touch his robe to receive and connect with his overflowing energy. Touching of garments also occurs today with Indian saints, and it must certainly have happened with Christian saints as well. I still remember being touched by the hands of my spiritual master Osho in India twenty years ago. Such an experience is never forgotten.

After the Meiji Emperor's poems were recited, Dr. Usui told the participants about where Reiki comes from and how it is used. He then used one or two case histories to illustrate his points. Afterward, the participants practiced the *Gassho* meditation and the *Joshin Kokyuu-Ho* breathing technique described later in this chapter. Then they healed each other.

The Reiki Techniques of Dr. Usui

As with meditation practice, the results of the techniques are not necessarily immediate. Or they may be immediate and then seem to fade away again. We may think they are wearing off. But, at the start, we are simply not used to the increased amount of energy flowing through our system. After a while, we no longer feel it as intensely. If it happens to you, keep going and practice each method for at least three months. If you do not have enough time to practice all of them, pick out one or two or three that touch your heart. Focus on them with your total energy. You will be rewarded greatly for your efforts.

If you have not yet learned these techniques, it is advisable to find someone in your area who teaches them. After all, people are the best teachers—not books.

My last book, *The Original Reiki Handbook of Dr. Mikao Usui*, discussed what I call the three pillars of Reiki. Dr. Usui said that the Reiki Ryoho (method of healing) is based on *gassho* (two hands coming together), *reiji* (indication of the spirit), *chiryo* (treatment), and the five Reiki principles.

What follows is a more detailed explanation of the terms and how the techniques are practiced, including their energetic or/and esoteric background.

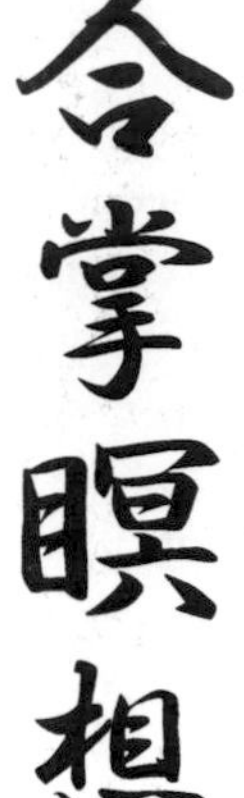

1. *Gassho Meiso:* The Gassho Meditation

The Japanese word *gassho* means "two hands coming together.

- Practice *gassho* by comfortably folding your hands in front of your heart center. Mr. Ogawa suggested that the hands should be held so that if you were to exhale through the nose the exiting breath would gently touch your fingertips. His suggestion shows the height at which to hold your hands.
- Inhale through your nose and exhale through your mouth during the course of this meditation. Common Qi Gong practice suggests that you rest your tongue on the roof of your mouth as you inhale; while exhaling, let your tongue drop to the bottom of your mouth. Positioning the tongue as described completes the circle of energy within the body and mind.
- Close your eyes and sit in a relaxed position, either on a chair or on the floor in the lotus or half-lotus position. Keep your back as straight as possible without straining it. If necessary, use support for your back. Leaning against the wall is also fine.

The experience of many people worldwide who meditate indicates that meditation is easiest when the spine is held erect. But you can certainly meditate sitting in a chair or lying down. Once you have gotten the knack of it, you can meditate anywhere and at any time with either closed or open eyes. Meditativeness then enters your every action, filling your life with serenity and grace.

If possible, leave your eyes closed the whole time in order to keep the energy within yourself. We have become accustomed to looking around and getting stimulated by visual impulses. The impulses lead to a train of thought that we automatically follow, leading us into a jungle of unconsciousness.

If you feel uncomfortable with your eyes closed, keep them open but unfocused and don't blink. After a few minutes, your eyes will begin to get teary, but keep going. When you have practiced a few times, you will be able to avoid blinking your eyes during the entire meditation. Blinking eyes and arising thoughts often go hand in hand. No blinking, no thinking! You can also use a blindfold to keep your eyes gently closed.

Let the breath enter your body on its own. There is no need to regulate it in any way. Just inhale deeply into your belly. If you don't know how to do this, either ask someone to show you or put one hand on your belly and try to breathe into the area you are touching. You will soon get the hang of it. Make it a point to practice ever day, and your breath will soon reach deeper and deeper into your belly. An exercise that will help you very quickly experience belly breathing is the Joshin Kokyuu-Ho technique described later.

The purpose of *gassho* meditation is to increase the energy of the practitioner and to put him or her into a meditative frame of mind. Practice it every day either in the morning or the evening (or both), alone or in a group, for twenty to thirty minutes.

The instructions for gassho meditation are simple: *Concentrate all of your attention on the point where both middle fingers touch and forget everything else.*

Our normal state of mind is absolute chaotic craziness. The trick is to first become aware of this craziness and then, without trying to make the craziness go away, turn the poison into nectar.

Osho told a beautiful tale about Mullah Nasruddin, a humorous character in mystic Islam whose stories are used to illustrate human nature:

> *In his garden Mullah had a beautiful apple tree that bore many delicious fruits. It was well known in his neighborhood, and many children sneaked into the garden to steal his apples when they became ripe. Every time the Mullah saw a child coming up to the apple tree, he would charge out of the house screaming and yelling at the offender. One day, a neighbor who had been watching the daily drama took the Mullah by the arm and said, "Mullah, you are such a peaceful man, and the tree in your garden yields so much more than you could possibly eat. Why do you chase the poor children away?"*
>
> *"Children," said Mullah, "are like thoughts. When you chase them away, you can be assured they will return."*

Keep this story in mind when you are meditating. Don't chase away the thoughts that cloud your mind's eye. Look at them, acknowledge them, and then bring your attention back to the point where the middle fingers meet. With the *gassho* meditation, we meditate and show our gratefulness to God or existence or whatever you call the ultimate principle by placing our hands in front of our hearts.

It has been our experience with hundreds of seminar participants that gassho meditation fits both the Eastern and the Western mind very well. Old and young, regardless of their background, enjoy it. One remark often shared with us is that the practice makes it easy for many of us to watch our internal dialogue and be less fidgety than usual.

In esoteric Buddhism the left hand represents the moon and the right hand stands for the sun.

Each finger represents one of the five elements:
The thumbs represent the Void.
The index fingers represent Air.
The middle fingers represent Fire.
The ring fingers represent Water.
The little fingers represent Earth.

According to esoteric Buddhism, the fingertips relate to certain qualities:
The thumbs represent discernment.
The index fingers represent operation.
The middle fingers represent perception.
The ring fingers represent reception.
The little fingers represent form.

From the standpoint of meditative science, the sun and moon and all the elements come together when we fold our hands. The circle is complete. Focusing our attention on the middle finger emphasizes the fire aspect of meditation—awareness burning the unconscious elements.

Your fingertips also are the home of many nerve endings and meridians. The meridian that ends in the middle finger is the pericardium meridian of the hand *(jueyin)*. It runs from the chest along the medial side of the arm, past the wrist, through the palm of the hand, and terminates in the tip of the middle finger. If your hands become tired while meditating, allow them to gently come down and rest in your lap. Keep focusing your attention on the point where the two middle fingers meet.

Technique 1—*Gassho Meiso:* The Meditation

1–3: *Sit and fold your hands together in a confortable position in front of your chest Focus your whole attention on the point where the two middle fingers meet and forget all the rest.*

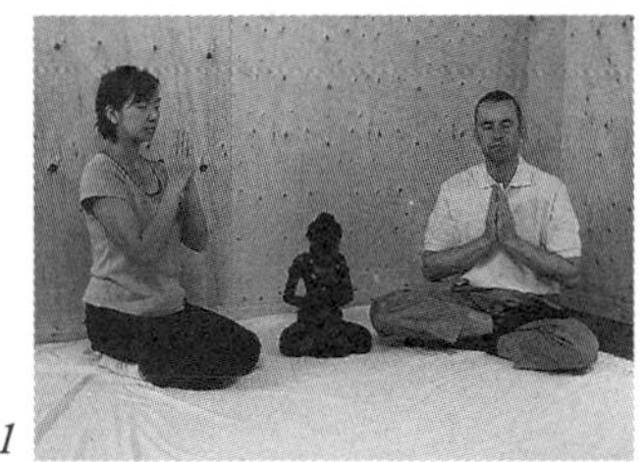

1

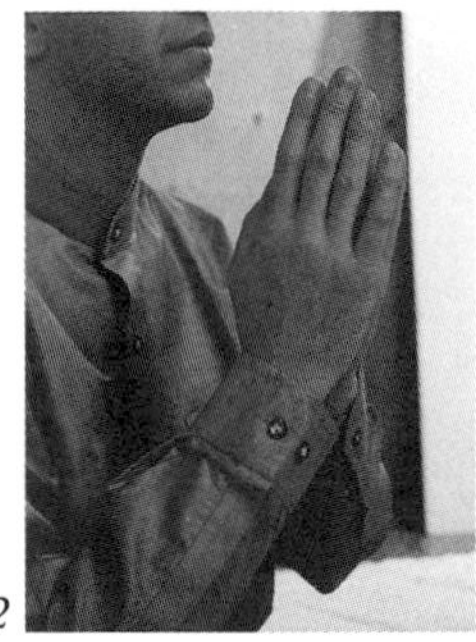

2

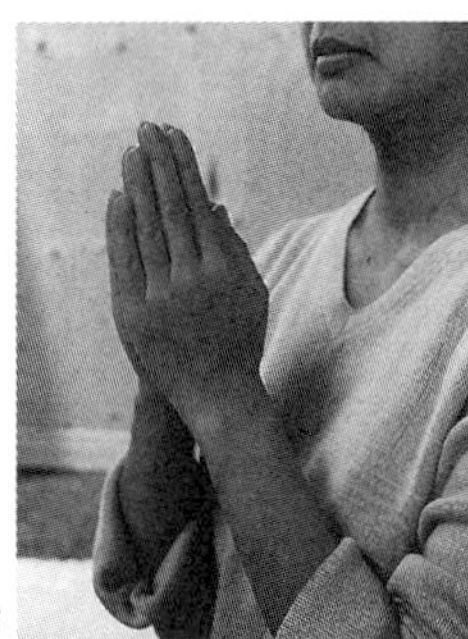

3

霊示

2. *Reiji-Ho:* The Indication of Reiki Energy

The Japanese word *Reiji* means "indication of the spirit," or indication of the Reiki energy in our case. In Hawayo Takata's diary, the technique is described as the "utmost secret in the energy science." She writes the word *Reiji-Ho* with an L (*Leiji-Ho)* instead of an R!

The technique teaches us to follow our intuition. We don't need to develop our intuition, as it is already bestowed upon us at birth as a divine gift. All we have to do is learn to listen to it and then follow it. We have all experienced many times not following our intuition—often our first impression. We frequently regret it later! The more I trust life and myself, the clearer my intuition becomes.

It may be very gratifying for the ego to think that we create our own reality and we manifest events and situations in our lives, but my experience has not confirmed this theory. Of course, we need to be open to receive abundance, but life ultimately takes its own course in spite of us. What we can learn is not to stop the flow, to step out of the way and let life live itself.

In the case of Reiki and the *Reiji* technique, letting life live itself means becoming a hollow bamboo for the energy to flow through, without regard to where, when, and how it may happen.

The instructions for this technique are simple and to the point:

- *Sit or stand in a comfortable position and close your eyes.*
- *Fold your hands in front of your heart and ask the energy to flow through you freely.*
- *Ask for the healing and well-being of your client on every level, whatever that may mean.*
- *Bring your folded hands up to the third eye and ask Reiki to guide your hands to wherever they are needed.*

Now wait and see what happens. You may be immediately guided to a certain area of the body. It can happen in many different ways. If you tend to be visually oriented, you may see a body part in front of your inner eye or the body part to be treated may "jump" out at you.

If you tend to be auditory, you may hear what part of the body you should first treat.

If you are the kinesthetic/feeling type, you may simply feel where you should touch your client. Some people feel the prompting within their own bodies.

Use all clues available to you. Use all your senses and knowledge of the body to tune in to your client. You may also tell your client to ask his or her body where it needs to be touched. Often it is quite obvious to see what is happening with someone's body by simply looking at the way it lays on the massage table in front of you. Check how the head is resting—is it straight or tilted to one side? Is the body twitching? Are the limbs straight or does one leg appear longer than the other? Is the spine twisted? If you can see a twist in the body but don't know where this tension is coming from, gently recreate that tension within your own body and feel where it is. For example, an imbalance in the left shoulder area could have its origin in the right lower back. When you have found the tense body part, treat it.

If you do not get a clear message with the *Reiji* technique right away, hold one or both of your hands over the client's crown chakra and tune into his or her energy body. If you still can't tell, use the *byosen* scanning method discussed later (see page 162-163). After years of training—or if you are already very skilled at listening to your intuition—you may be able to "see" ailments in your clients just by looking at them.

When your client lies on the massage table in front of you and your hands are guided to the abdominal cavity, it may not be clear which vital organ is attracting your hands. Ms. Koyama suggests that the easiest way to check is by simply asking yourself: Is it the gall bladder, is it the descending colon, is it the pancreas, etc.? Then let your hands answer your mind's questions.

You have to discover for yourself how this answer is given to you. It may be a tingling in your hands, a certain warmth, a magnetic feeling, or simply knowing.

The idea that we are separate from the rest of the world is an illusion. We must realize that wisdom is infinite and available to all of us. We only have to learn to tap into the collective knowledge of humanity. With the *Reiji-Ho* approach, all you need to do is ask.

Once you have mastered the art of *Reiji-Ho* for healing, you can expand it into other areas of your life, such as creativity.

Technique 2—*Reiji-Ho:* The Reiki Prayer

1: *Fold your hands in front of your chest and ask the energy to flow through you freely.*
2: *Ask for the healing and well-being of your client on every level.*
3: *Bring your folded hands up to the third eye and ask Reiki to guide your hands to wherever they are needed.*
4: *Follow your hands and begin the treatment.*

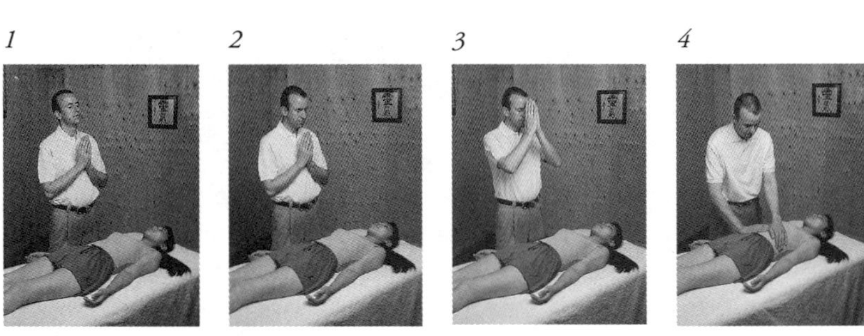

1 *2* *3* *4*

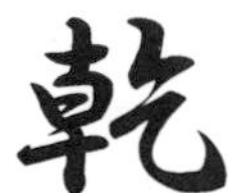
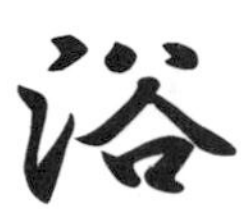

3. *The Kenyoku-Technique:* Dry Bathing

The Japanese word *kenyoku* means "dry bathing." *Kenyoku* purifies body and soul, instead of the old-fashioned way of splashing ice cold water over oneself (traditional Japanese method). It strengthens your energy and helps you to detach from your clients, situations, thoughts, and emotions. It brings you into the present moment. Many times during the day we get lost in our own minds, thoughts, problems, joys, and other emotions. Or we get drawn into those of our fellow human beings. Neither situation helps us on the path to self-discovery. When we are drawn into our own daydreams or those of another person, we lose ourselves and enter into an automatic train of thought, which is absolutely involuntary. It is like a monkey swinging from one branch to the next, ad infinitum. We miss out on the present moment, the only time that really exists. It is difficult for us to break the identification with our thoughts because it keeps us engaged in mental or emotional activities.

In the course of our Reiki research, we have come across three ways of practicing kenyoku.

Dr. Usui was said to have taught it like this (version 1):

- Place your right hand on the left side of your chest, over the collarbone. Now stroke down gently across your chest to the right hipbone. Do the same with your left hand, starting on the right side of your chest, over the collarbone. Stroke down gently toward your left hipbone. Repeat the motion with your right hand.
- Now use your right hand to gently stroke from your left wrist over the open palm of your left hand, past your fingertips. Then use your left hand to gently stroke from your right wrist over the open palm of your right hand, past your fingertips. (Some Reiki schools suggest repeat this motion once more with the right hand.)

A variation is also widely practiced today (version 2):

- Place your right hand on the left side of your chest, over the collarbone. Now stroke down gently across your chest to the right hipbone. Do the same with your left hand, starting on the right side of your chest, above the collarbone. Stroke down gently towards your left hipbone. Repeat the motion with your right hand.
- Now place your right hand on your left shoulder and stroke down gently over the outside of your arm and the outside of your hand, past your fingertips. Do the same stroke with your left hand over the outside of your right arm. (Some Reiki schools suggest repeat this motion once more with the right hand.)

Here is a further variation (version 3):

- Place your right hand on the left side of your chest, over the collarbone. Now stroke down gently across your chest to the right hipbone. Do the same with your left hand, starting on the right side of your chest, above the collarbone. Stroke down gently toward your left hipbone. Repeat the motion with your right hand.
- Now place your right hand on your left shoulder and stroke down gently over the inside of your left arm and the palm of your left hand, past your fingertips. Do the same stroke with your left hand over the inside of your right arm. (Some Reiki schools suggest repeat this motion once more with the right hand.) A former Buddhist monk taught me this technique. In his school of Reiki, they add a *Gassho* at the end of the *Kenyoku* technique. If this feels good to you, include it.

If the circumstances don't allow you to go through the physical motions of the technique, do it in your imagination.

I personally practice technique number three. However, I suggest that you find the best technique for you by practicing it yourself. When all is said and done, you are your own best teacher.

Technique 3—*Kenyoku:* Dry Bathing (version 1)

1–6: *Place your right hand on the left side of your chest, over the collarbone. Stroke down gently across your chest to the right hipbone. Do the same with your left hand, starting on the right side of your chest, over the collarbone. Stroke down gently toward your left hipbone. Repeat the motion with your right hand.*

7–12: *Now use your right hand to gently stroke from your* ***left wrist*** *over the* ***open palm*** *of your left hand, past your fingertips. Then use your left hand to gently stroke from your* ***right wrist*** *over the open palm of your right hand, past your fingertips. (Some Reiki schools suggest repeat this motion once more with the right hand.)*

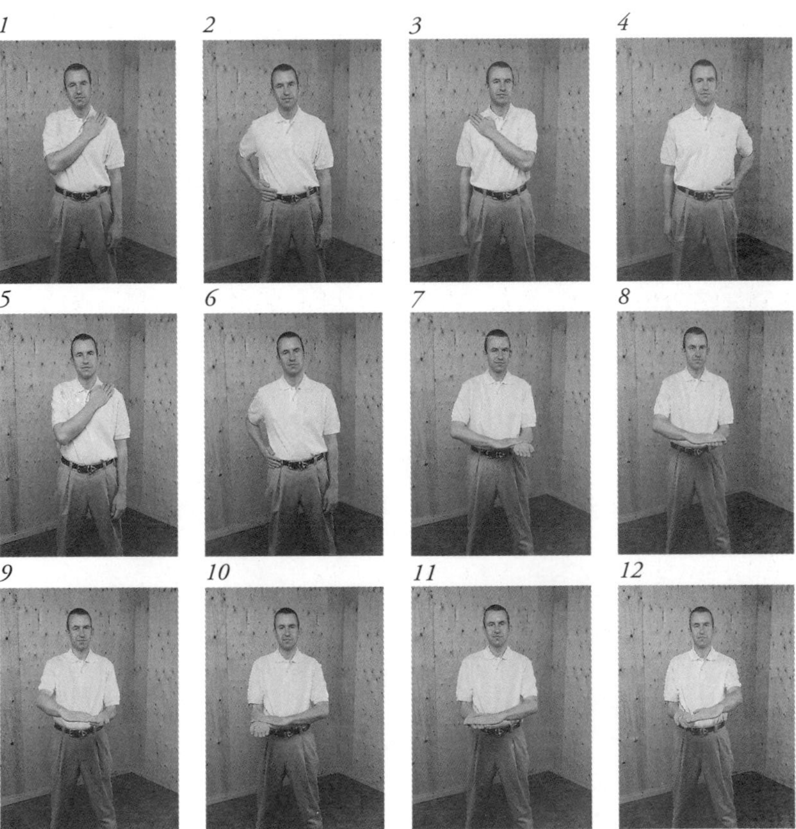

Technique 3—*Kenyoku:* Dry Bathing (version 2)

1–6: *Place your right hand on the left side of your chest, over the collarbone. Now stroke down gently across your chest to the right hipbone. Do the same with your left hand, starting on the right side of your chest, above the collarbone. Stroke down gently towards your left hipbone. Repeat the motion with your right hand.*

7–12: *Now place your right hand on your* ***left shoulder*** *and stroke down gently over the* ***outside of your arm*** *and the outside of your hand, past your fingertips. Do the same stroke with your left hand from your* ***right shoulder*** *over the* ***outside of your right arm****. (Some Reiki schools suggest repeat this motion once more with the right hand.)*

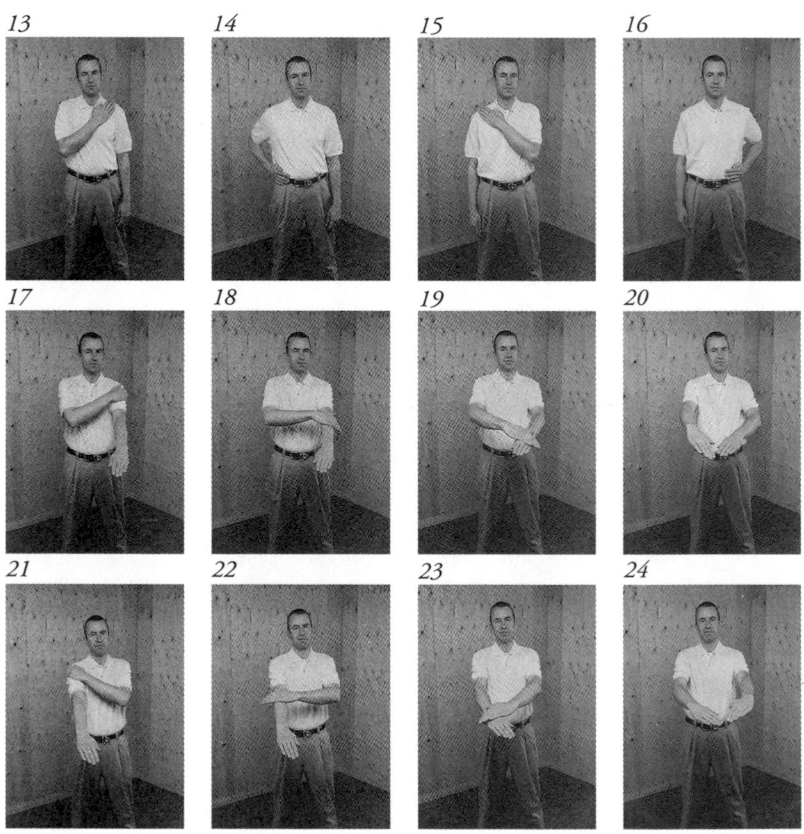

Technique 3—*Kenyoku:* Dry Bathing (version 3)

13–16: *Place your right hand on the left side of your chest, over the collarbone. Now stroke down gently across your chest to the right hipbone. Do the same with your left hand, starting on the right side of your chest, above the collarbone. Stroke down gently toward your left hipbone. Repeat the motion with your right hand.*

17–24: *Now place your right hand on your* ***left shoulder*** *and stroke down gently over the* ***inside of your left arm*** *and the palm of your left hand, past your fingertips.*

29–32: *Do the same stroke with your left hand from your* ***right shoulder*** *over the* ***inside of your right arm.*** *(Some Reiki schools suggest repeat this motion once more with the right hand.)*

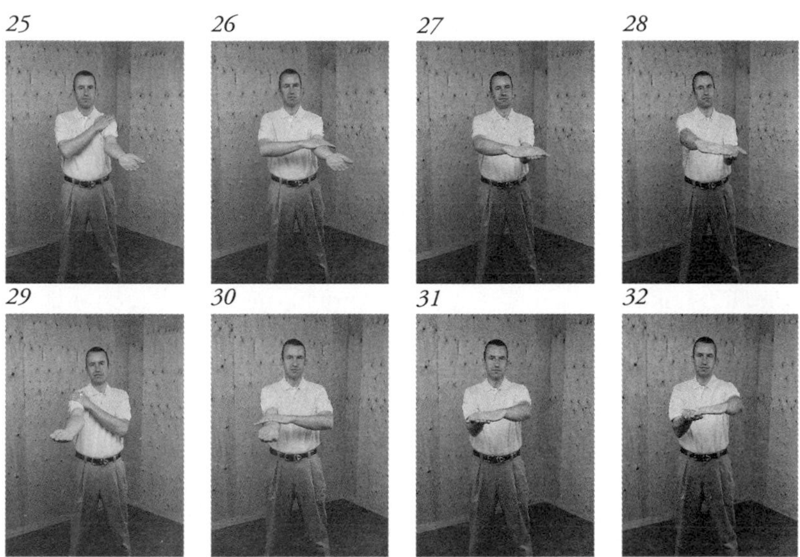

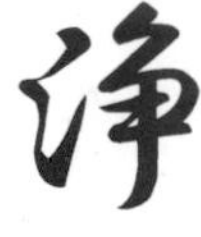

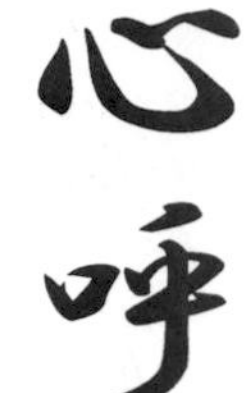

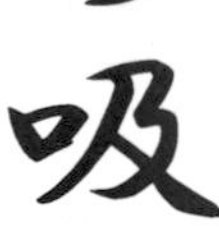

4. *Joshin Kokyuu-Ho:* The Breathing Technique

The Japanese phrase *Joshin Kokyuu-Ho* means "breathing exercise to purify the spirit." It is a breathing technique to strengthen your energy. It will teach you to consciously draw in energy from the cosmos and collect it in your *tanden**. Then you can let the energy flow out through your hands:

- Inhale through your nose and imagine drawing Reiki energy into your body through the crown chakra. Pull the energy down into your tanden. When the breath reaches your tanden, keep it there for a few seconds without straining yourself. Find your own rhythm. Visualize how the breath is expanding and permeating your entire body. Then exhale through your mouth and imagine the energy flowing out through your fingertips, your hand chakras, the tips of your toes, and your foot chakras.

The technique magnifies your Reiki energy and helps you feel like a piece of hollow bamboo—a clear channel for energy. When practicing this it, you will realize that energy does not belong to us. It is simply the all-pervading force that makes everything pulsate with life. With practice, you will find that the forces you thought to be your own personal energy melt and merge with the cosmic energy within your body-mind system. Then it becomes exceedingly difficult to draw the line between where the universe ends and "I" begin.

Teaching the technique is a great pleasure, especially to Reiki beginners. Beginners are frequently so certain that even though everybody else can sense, see, or feel the energy they won't because they are particularly insensitive. In my experience, no one has been able to resist the technique!

If you are unsure about the exact location of the tanden, you will be able to find it with the help of the following exercise, which is

* Chinese: *tantien* or *dantien*, located two or three fingers below the navel.

widely used in martial-arts traditions for centering. (Some people say that the tanden is identical with the second chakra. Others believe that it is a center in its own right, independent of the chakra system.)

Contraindication: Not to be used by someone with high blood pressure or during pregnancy. If you feel light-headed at any time while practicing, discontinue the exercise immediately.

How to find the tanden:

- Stand in a comfortable position with your feet shoulder-width apart.
- Take a few deep breaths.
- Release all of the tension in your body and think of something pleasant.
- Let your mouth open slightly.
- Rest your tongue on the roof of your mouth as you inhale. Breathe in through your nose. When exhaling through your mouth, let your tongue naturally come down and rest at the bottom of your mouth.
- Bend your knees in slow motion while focusing your attention on your lower abdomen.
- Do the steps very, very slowly.
- Suddenly, you will become aware of a point in your lower abdomen, two or three fingers below your navel. It is where your life force dwells, the center of your being.
- Now begin with the breathing technique.
- It may help to put one or both of your hands on your lower abdomen and breathe into the spot you are touching.

We not only breathe through our lungs, taking in a mixture of gases commonly called "air." Modern medical science understands that each cell is able to breathe. So we would die if that ability were suspended for a certain period of time, as in the case of severe burns. All esoteric disciplines know that we "inhale" energy as Ki, chi, prana, or whatever you may call it both through our lungs and through the skin, our largest organ.

Some fakirs of the past and "breatharians" of modern times have been known to sustain their bodies without eating. (Certain fakirs even managed without breathing for a long time.) It is a well-known fact that people in a good physical condition can easily fast for as long as six weeks without complications. (Please don't try it by yourself—fasting should be done only under the supervision of a capable health-care practitioner.) To keep the body alive, we only need a minimal amount of food. The actions we perform are what require us to supply the body with the necessary fuel.

I personally don't see any great value in not eating or breathing. We are perfectly fine the way we are, even with our lungs filled with air and our stomach full of food! The important point is that breathing exercises and fasting can help us more efficiently use the subtle energies surrounding us. The more we grow on the spiritual path, the greater amounts of subtle fuel we need to keep a clear mind and a pure heart.

To draw in the subtle energy, we need to breathe deeply into the belly, all the way down to the tanden. I discussed breathing into the tanden in greater detail in the chapter on "The Journey from the Head to the Heart and from the Heart to the Belly" on page 90.

Technique 4—*Joshin Kokyuu-Ho*: The Breathing Technique to Purify the Spirit

Preliminary exercise:

1: *Stand in a comfortable position, feet shoulder-width apart.*

2: *Take a few deep breaths. Release all the tension in your body and think of something pleasant. Let your mouth open slightly. Rest your tongue on the roof of your mouth as you inhale. Breathe in through your nose. When exhaling through your mouth, let your tongue naturally come down and rest at the bottom of your mouth.*

3: *Bend your knees in slow motion while focusing your attention on your lower abdomen. Do so very, very slowly. Suddenly, you will become aware of a point in your lower abdomen, two or three fingers below your navel.*

Main exercise:

Inhale through your nose and imagine drawing Reiki energy into your body through the crown chakra. Pull the energy down to your tanden. When the breath reaches your tanden, keep it there for a few seconds without straining yourself. Visualize how this breath is expanding and permeating your entire body. Then exhale through your mouth and imagine the energy flowing out through your fingertips, your hand chakras, the tips of your toes, and your foot chakras.

1

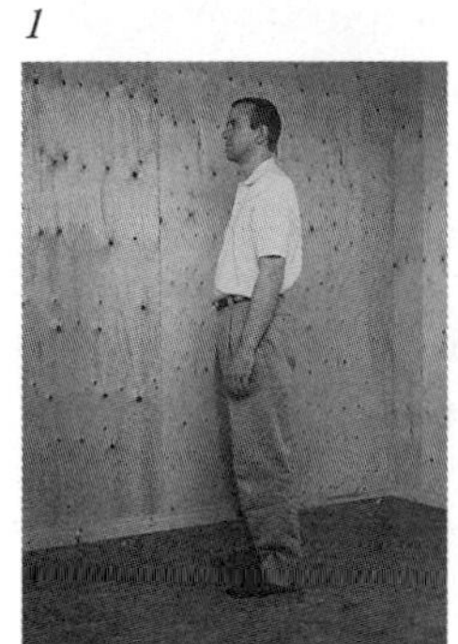

2

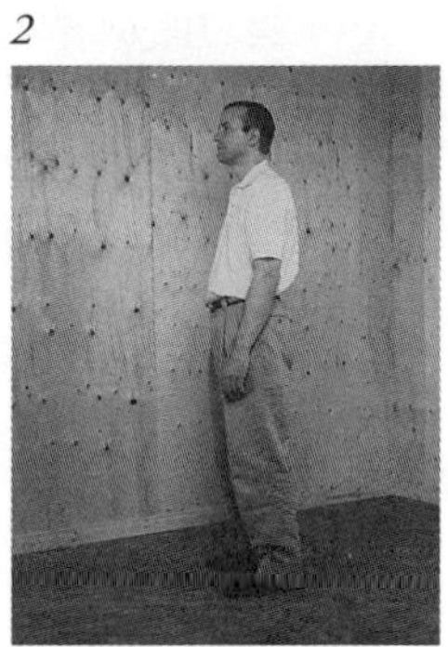

3

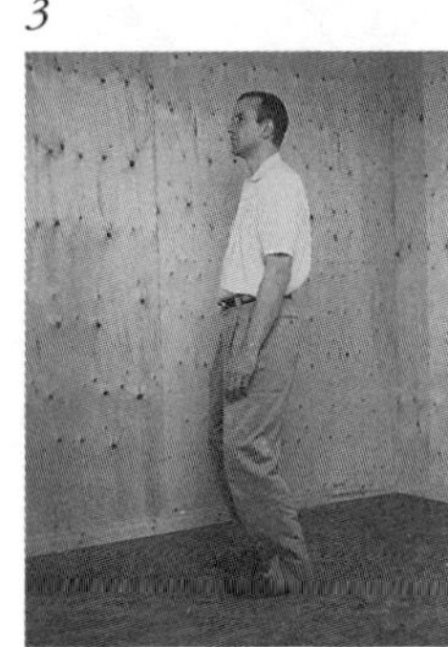

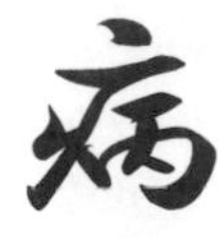

5. *Byosen:* The Scanning Technique

The Japanese word *byo* means "sick" and the word *sen* means "line."

- Fold your hands in the *gassho* position in front of your heart. Pray that the energy will come through you and guide you to the body part that needs treatment. If your hands are pulled to a specific body part immediately, follow them. If not, place your dominant hand above the client's crown chakra and attune yourself to it. If you still don't feel guided, scan the front and back of the body in slow downward movements.

You may feel a tingling sensation in your hands. It may be a feeling of heat, magnetism, pressure, or just a deep knowing that you have found the right spot. Maybe you "see" the right body part or you may "hear" it. You're not going nuts! It is normal for an auditory person to "hear voices" and for a visual person to have "slight hallucinations." Just be as aware as possible.

When you touch the body part that has indicated itself to you, you may experience an uncomfortable feeling in your hand(s), which may move up your arm(s) and sometimes even into your shoulder(s). Instead of taking your hands off the body to avoid the unpleasant sensation, stay with it. Wait for the sensation to trace back down your arm and out of your hands. Then let yourself be guided to the next position.

According to Ms. Koyama, the unpleasantness is caused by the positive Reiki energy directed to a negatively charged body part, creating the sensation called *hibiki*. If you continue sending Reiki, eventually the unpleasant sensation will trace back down into your fingertips and out of them.

If it is not possible (or advisable) to touch the sick part directly with your hand(s), you can hold your hands above the body part.

In one of my seminars, someone shared that he and his colleagues had discovered that, with training, it is possible to feel the particular *byosen* of HIV-positive patients in the left upper region of the chest below the collarbone. I have not had any personal experience in treating HIV-positive patients, but the insight may be helpful.

Technique 5—*Byosen:* Scanning

1–6: *Scan the front and back of the body in slow downward movements.*

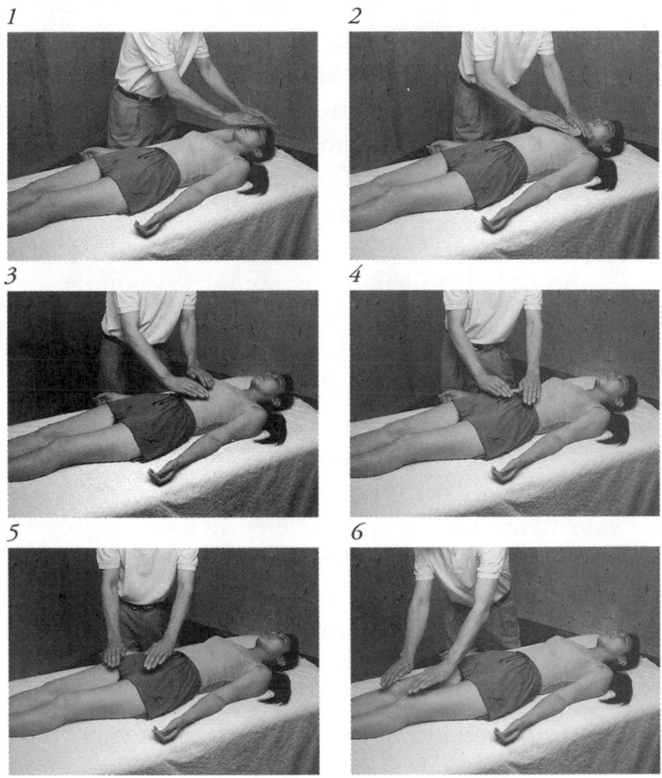

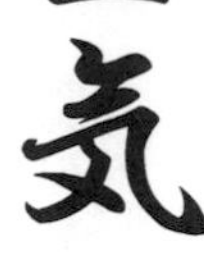
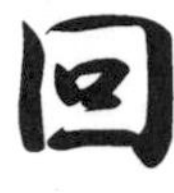

6. *Reiki Mawashi:* Reiki Current Group Exercise

The Japanese word *mawashi* means "current." In the exercise a current of Reiki energy is passed through a group of practitioners similarly to how many of you practice Reiki in your meetings.

- In the group sit in a circle and hold your hands a few inches above/below the hands of your neighbors—so that the left hand extends to the neighbor on the left and the right hand to the neighbor on the right. Turn your left hand upward and your right hand downward. The teacher begins the flow of energy, sending the energy to his or her left. The recipient receives the energy from his or her right hand, lets it flow through his or her body, and passes it on to the next individual through his or her left hand. Practice for ten minutes.

I don't know if it matters which direction the energy is sent. Theories abound on the earth's magnetism; some people claim the exercise should be done to the right above the equator and to the left below the equator. Theories are great, but they should not limit us in any way. Experiment with both ways to see what feels most natural to you and your Reiki friends. Our preferences are probably rooted in what we are accustomed to. I think both ways will work anywhere on the planet—and maybe beyond! In any event once we have learned to direct energy, it should not matter whether we direct it to the left, right, above, or below.

The energy of a group often exceeds the sum of the energy of the participants, and spontaneous healing on all levels may occur. I usually perform the exercise for ten to fifteen minutes in my seminars. Reiki Two or Reiki Three practitioners may use the Second or Third Degree Reiki symbols while practicing it.

Technique 6—*Reiki Mawashi:* Reiki Group Exercise

1: *Sit in a circle and hold your hands a few inches above/below the hands of your neighbors. Your left hand is facing up, the right one is facing down.*

2: *Sit in a circle and hold the hands of your neighbors. Your left hand is facing up, the right one is facing down*

1

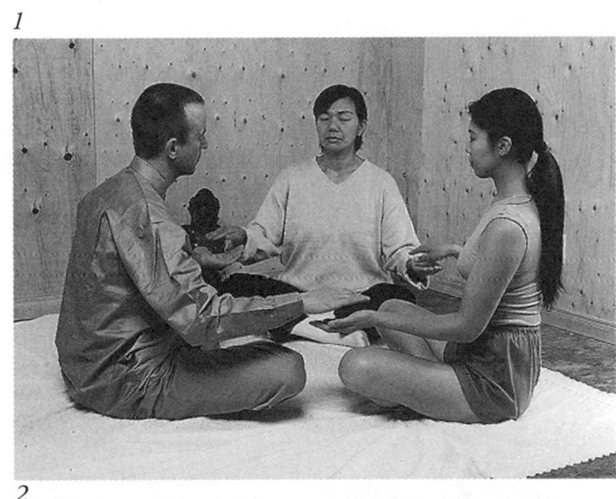

2

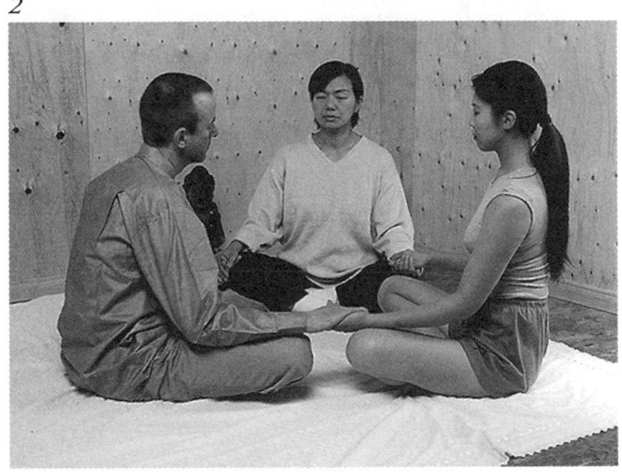

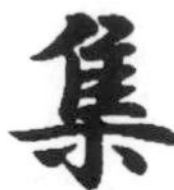
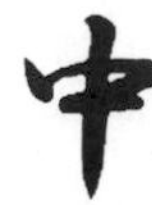
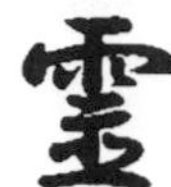
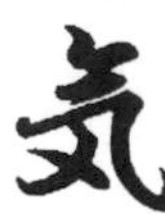

7. *Shu Chu-Reiki:* Concentrated Reiki Group Exercise

The Japanese word *shu chu* literally means "concentrated." This technique can be practiced in a group or at a Reiki meeting.

- All group members give energy to one group member, wishing and praying for the other person's happiness and health.

  First Degree Reiki practitioners lay their hands directly on the client and Second Degree Reiki practitioners may use the Reiki symbols. Second degree practitioners can also use distance (absentee) healing.

The exercise can be an intense experience for the client, so it is not advisable for many practitioners to so treat clients who are emotionally unstable. If the practicing group is very large, do it for one or two minutes each.

In large groups, it may not be possible for everyone to touch the person to be treated. So what we do is form several rows of healers around the massage table. The first row touches the "patient" directly and the second and third rows touch the shoulders of the people in the first and second row. The energy thus flows and surges through everyone participating in the healing and finally reaches the "patient." It is a wonderful experience for everyone involved.

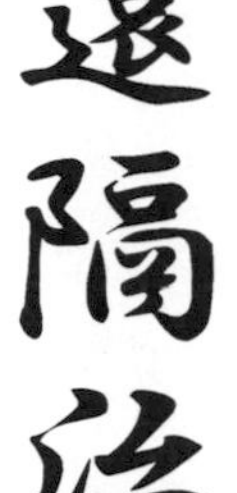

8. *Enkaku Chiryo* (*Shashin Chiryo*): Distant Healing Techniques

Dr. Usui apparently was very fond of distant healing. He used it even if the recipient was just in the next room. He taught this technique during *Okuden Koki* (the last part of *Okuden*, our Second Degree). The Japanese word *enkaku* means "sending" and the work *chiryo* means "treatment." The method has also been known in Japan as *shashin chiryo* or "photographic treatment."

As many distant healing methods probably exist as there are Reiki practitioners. All the methods are designed to help us focus our minds.

- If possible, use a photograph of the recipient. Write his or her name and date of birth on the back. If you have been asked to send energy on behalf of someone you don't personally know, try to gather as much additional information as possible and write it on the photograph as well. You will then better focus your energy. When using a photograph, it is easier to treat parts of the body that are usually not as accessible.
- If you don't have a picture of the recipient, draw with your hand an idol representing the other person on one of your fingers or knees and use that. It does not matter which finger or which knee you use.

Some Western Reiki teachers say you should not touch your own body when sending distant Reiki because you might send your own ailments to the other person. I find the idea quite amusing. Please don't worry about it. When you use your own body to send energy to another person, you simply use it to focus your mind.

It is not advisable to send energy to a person who has not specifically asked you for it. Reiki energy doesn't harm anyone, but it is important to respect other people's personal space and not interfere with their freedom even if this would happen for his/her own good.

Technique 8—*Enkaku Chiryo (Shashin Chiryo):* Distant Healing

1–2: *Draw an idol representing the other person on your finger.*
3–4: *Draw an idol representing the other person on your knee.*
5: *When using a photograph, it is easier to treat parts of the body that are usually not as accessible.*

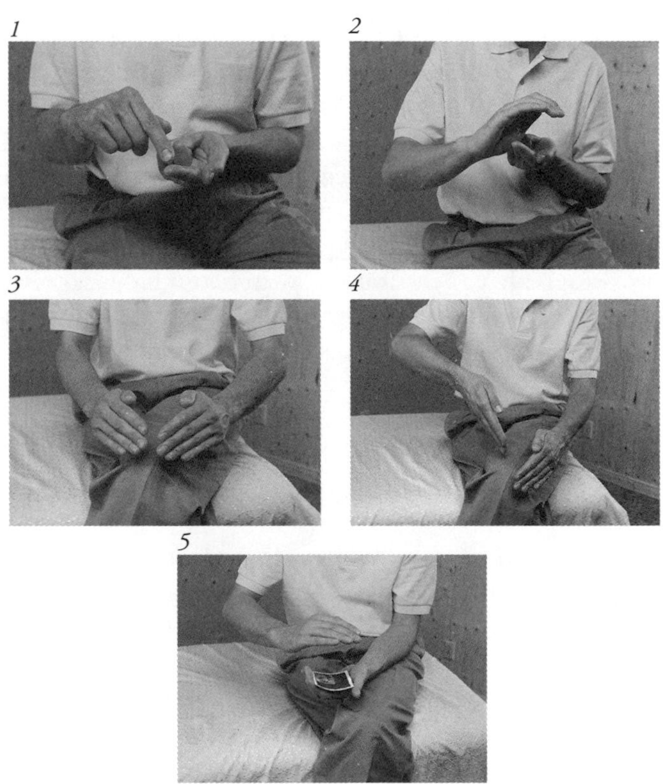

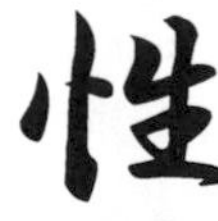

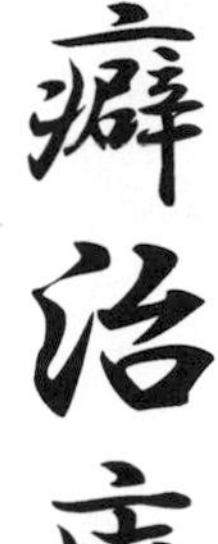

9. *Seiheki Chiryo:* Habit-Healing Technique

The Japanese word *seiheki* means "habit" and the word *chiryo* means "treatment." The technique is used for treating habits, especially what we would call "bad" habits. Many people have learned the technique known as the deprogramming technique in Western Reiki. The deprogramming technique is a sophisticated version of the original technique (as described in my book, *Reiki Fire*). It involves the use of Reiki symbols, but the technique discussed here doesn't. If you are working on yourself, make an affirmation. If you are working with clients, help them make affirmations. Remember that affirmations must be short, precise, and positive. They should be in the present tense and in the words of the person who will use it. Also bear in mind that an affirmation should never be limiting in any way.

In order to find out what people really want in their lives, you need to take your time. Our desires often have deeper meanings not initially obvious.

Here are the instructions:

- Place your nondominant hand (for instance the left hand if you are right-handed) on the forehead of the client (or your own forehead) and your dominant hand on the back of the head. Keep your hands there for two or three minutes while you intensely repeat the affirmation in your mind. Then, ceasing to think of the affirmation, remove your nondominant hand from the forehead and simply give Reiki to the recipient with your dominant hand still resting on the back of the head.

Dr. Usui supposedly used the five Reiki principles and the Meiji Emperor's poems with technique. Instead of making an affirmation, he would repeat the principles when touching the other person's forehead and back of the head.

Technique 9—*Seiheki Chiryo:* Habit-Healing

1: *Place your nondominant hand on the forehead of the client (or your own forehead at the self-treatment) and your dominant hand on the back of the head. Keep your hands there for two or three minutes while you intensely repeat the affirmation in your mind.*

2: *Then, ceasing to think of the affirmation, remove your nondominant hand from the forehead and simply give Reiki to the recipient with your dominant hand still resting on the back of the head.*

1

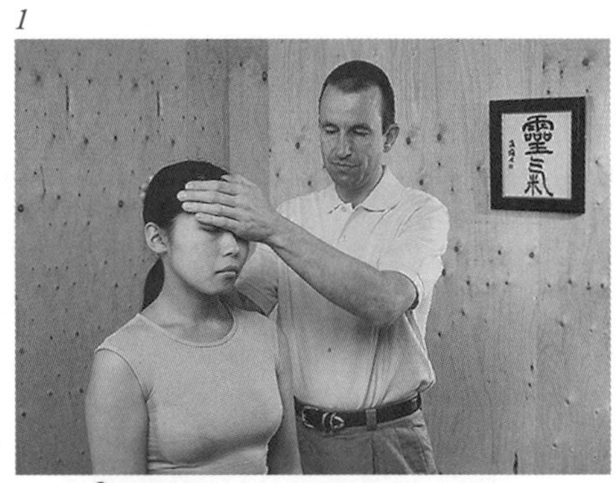

2

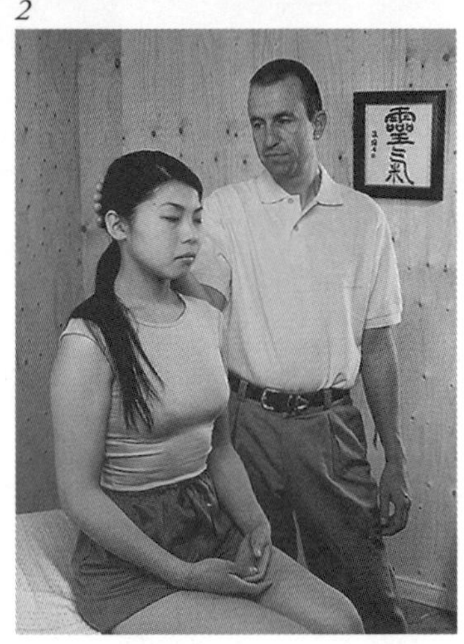

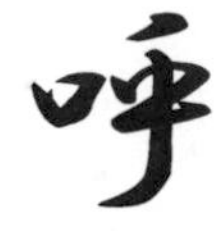
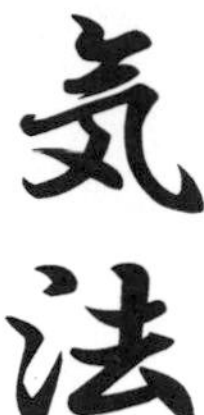

10. *Koki-Ho:* Healing with the Breath

As mentioned earlier, we inhale a mixture of gases and energy. The energy is obviously given off as we exhale. Dr. Usui reportedly said that if you feel hot while giving a Reiki treatment, you will be able to use both your breath and your eyes for administering Reiki. It helps to learn Reiki Two in order to work with the breath. Mr. Ogawa taught us Koki-Ho in the following way:

- Inhale and pull the breath down into your tanden. Hold it there for a few seconds and draw the power symbol on the roof of your mouth with your tongue.
- Now exhale and breathe the symbol onto the body part to be treated. You can thus work on the physical body, in the aura, and with photographs (distant healing). It is also helpful to visualize the power symbol as you exhale. (If you smoke and work with your breath on a client, make sure to use breath-freshener beforehand.)

You may also experiment with contracting the anal sphincter or Hui Yin* point while you work with the breath. Be aware that a breath treatment can be a powerful experience. In one of our seminars, Walter blew me away and I had a hard time coming back and leading the group!

---

* In China, the anal sphincter muscle Hui Yin, located between the sexual organs and the anus, is considered to be one of the most important energy gateways. Because the life energy can easily flow out of the body at this point, the contraction of the anal sphincter muscle is practiced in the Taoist tradition.
The goal of this contraction is to keep the life energy within the body and let it rise in the spinal column to the higher energy centers.
This exercise also prevents prostate problems.

Technique 10—*Koki-Ho:* Healing with the Breath

1–4: *Inhale and pull the breath down into your tanden. Hold it there for a few seconds and draw the power symbol on the roof of your mouth with your tongue. Then exhale and breathe the power symbol onto the body part to be treated.*

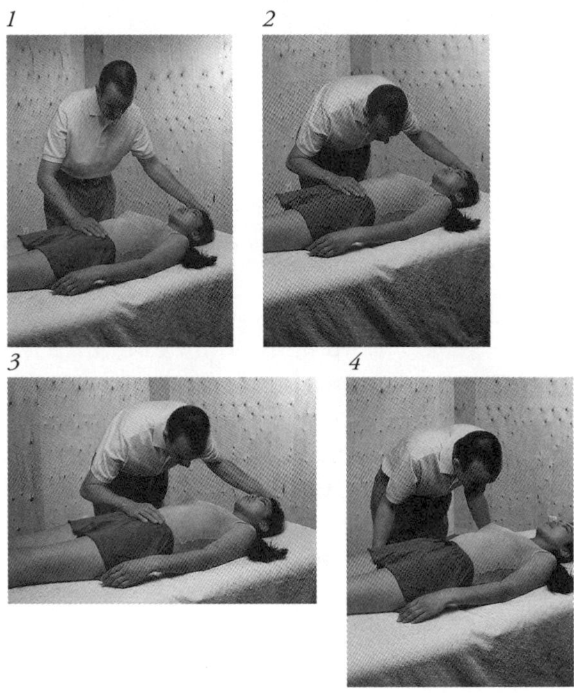

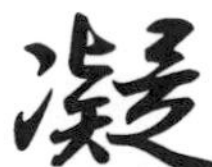

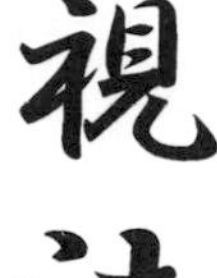

11. *Gyoshi-Ho:* Healing with the Eyes

The Japanese word *gyoshi* means "staring." In his handbook, Dr. Usui wrote that energy radiates from all parts of the body, mostly from the hands, eyes, and breath of the initiate. We are accustomed to throw our energy through our eyes, but this technique teaches us to actually use it. In order to heal, we must first relax our eyes and unfocus them. Staring is aggressive, and an aggressive look does not heal—it intrudes.

It may be helpful to first practice the technique with an object such as a flower (see photograph on page 174.)

- Hold the flower in your hand or place it one or two feet away from you on a table at the height of your eyes. Unfocus your eyes by first relaxing them and then looking at the flower as if you were looking through it or behind it. After a moment, you will notice that your field of vision has become peripheral. You can now see almost 180 degrees!
- Then look at the flower and let the image come to you, instead of sending the arrows of your visual attention toward it. After a while, you may become aware of a very subtle form of breathing that happens through your eyes, connected with the inhalation and exhalation. Practice the exercise for ten minutes every day until you feel comfortable using it to treat a human.

Here are the instructions for healing with your eyes:

- For a few minutes, look with a soft focus at the body part you want to treat. While you look at the other person, let the image of the individual enter your eyes instead of "actively looking" at him or her. Notice how a circle of energy between you and the other person is created when you let the energy of this individual enter your eyes. You may want to project the Reiki symbols onto the part of the body you want to treat.

For those of you who enjoy the technique and would like to experiment further, you can practice the following Hindu meditation technique.

It is called *Tratak* meditation:

- Sit in a comfortable position for forty-five to sixty minutes and stare at a candle. Don't blink your eyes. After a few minutes, your eyes will begin to tear. Keep staring at the flame. With a little practice, you will be able to do this for one hour. Your consciousness will become as sharp and focused as a laser beam!

Tratak can also be practiced with a photograph or statue of an enlightened one. You can do it with a partner sitting opposite you, with your own image in a mirror, or in darkness in a completely darkened room. Practicing with a flame may make you fiery. If that is uncomfortable for you, it will be better to do it without a candle, staring at darkness instead.

Technique 11—*Gyoshi-Ho:* Healing with the Eyes

Preliminary exercise:

1: *Look at a flower and let the image come to you.*

2: *Focus at the body part you want to treat for some minutes. While you look at the other person, let the image of the other individual enter your eyes instead of "actively looking" at him or her.*

1

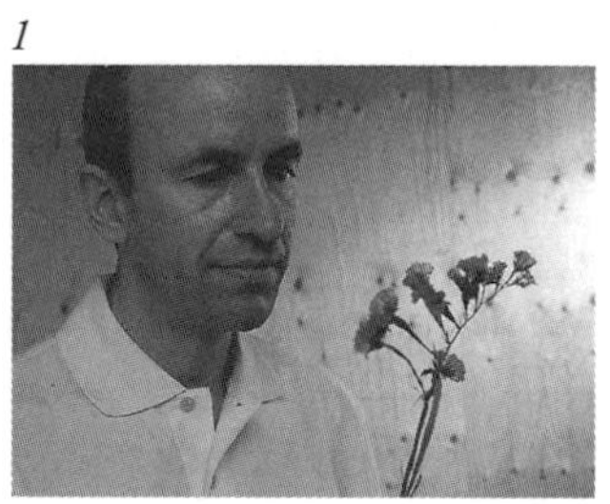

2

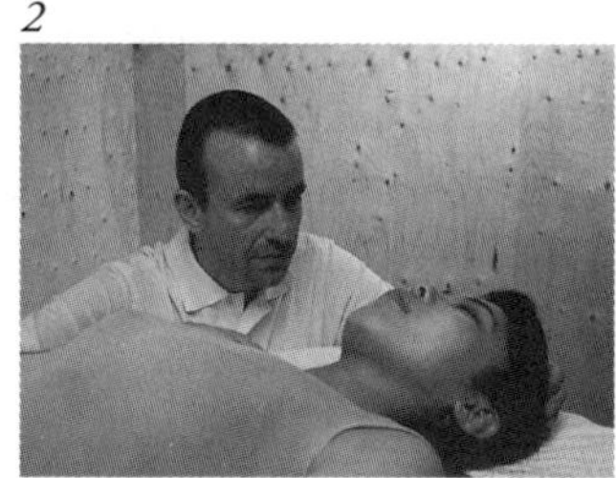

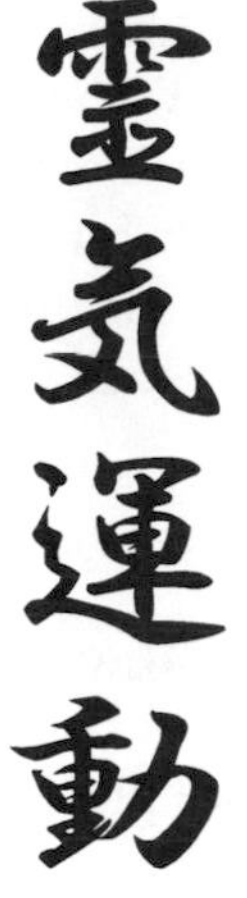

12. *Reiki Undo:* Reiki Exercise

The Japanese word *undo* means "exercise," and it refers to letting the body move without any restrictions. I was told that Ms. Koyama introduced the exercise to the Usui Reiki Ryoho. The technique is used all over the world and in many different cultures and traditions. In China, it is employed as part of Qi Gong training. In Indonesia, it is part of the *Subud* practice and is called *Latihan* in India.

Chetna came across something similar almost twenty years ago called *Katsugen Undo*. At that time as today it is taught by the *Noguchi Seitai* [26] group.

The instructions for Reiki Undo are very simple:
Find a place in your house where it is safe for you to roll around for twenty to thirty minutes so no one will disturb you. Make sure no sharp edges or furniture could hurt you.

- Start with *Gassho* and say in your mind, "Reiki exercise start!" Inhale deeply and when you exhale, let go completely. If you are practicing with a partner, touch his or her shoulders from behind and allow your body to move whatever way it wants to.
- Inhale deeply and let go as much as you can while you are exhaling. After taking a few deep breaths, your body will probably begin to move. If the movement doesn't come easily to you, be patient and don't create anything. Continue doing the exercise on a daily basis for at least three months.
- It may be difficult for you to let go completely and allow your body to move by itself. You may be clinging to the idea that you are an adult who shouldn't act like a child. Let go of the concept for the next twenty minutes and give yourself total freedom to behave like a child again.
- You may feel self-conscious, but no one is watching you. Think of nothing in particular. Take a little vacation from your adult self. If sounds come out of your mouth, don't restrict them. If thoughts and feelings come up, acknowledge and feel them. Don't hold back.

- It is quite likely that you will start to yawn, burp, and pass gas. Your eyes may begin to tear. (Sounds like fun, doesn't it?) Don't hold anything back for now—just let the body cleanse itself. It knows what to do and how to do it. We usually have the bad habit of restricting our own healing. Although certain restrictions may be appropriate in our day-to-day interactions with others, let it all go for now.
- Continue until the movements come to a complete stop.

Chetna learned the following technique from the *Noguchi Seitai* group many years ago. It is wonderful for getting your autonomic nervous system going. We could say that it "primes the pump" (see photographs 1-7 on page 177):

- Make a slight fist with both your hands, putting your thumbs inside them. Don't strain. Stretch out both arms straight in front of you. Now inhale deeply through your nose. While rigorously exhaling through your mouth, pull both arms toward you and tighten all of your muscles as tight as you can. When all of the air has escaped from your lungs and your arms are next to your body (with the fists somewhere near your shoulders), let go completely. Let your arms fall to your sides and allow your lungs to fill with air on their own. Repeat this exercise three to five times and then continue with *Reiki Undo*. You will know when the pump is primed.

In our seminars we practice Reiki Undo with the entire group if we have a safe environment that allows us to all sit together in a "train" (see photographs on page 178). One group participant remarked after the experience that the feeling of practicing *Reiki Undo* in a group came the closest to what she had experienced at Woodstock in 1969!

Technique 12—*Reiki Undo:* Reiki Exercise (Preliminary Exercise, Priming the Pump)

1–7: *With both hands, make a slight fist and put your thumb into it. Don't strain. Stretch out both arms straight in front of you. Now inhale deeply through your nose. While rigorously exhaling through your mouth, pull both arms toward your and tighten all of your muscles as tight as you can. When all the air has escaped from your lungs and your arms are next to your body (with the fists somewhere near your shoulders), let go completely. Let your arms fall to your sides and allow your lungs to fill with air on their own. Repeat the exercise three to five times and then continue with Reiki Undo (7-12 self-practice or 13-24 practice with a partner).*

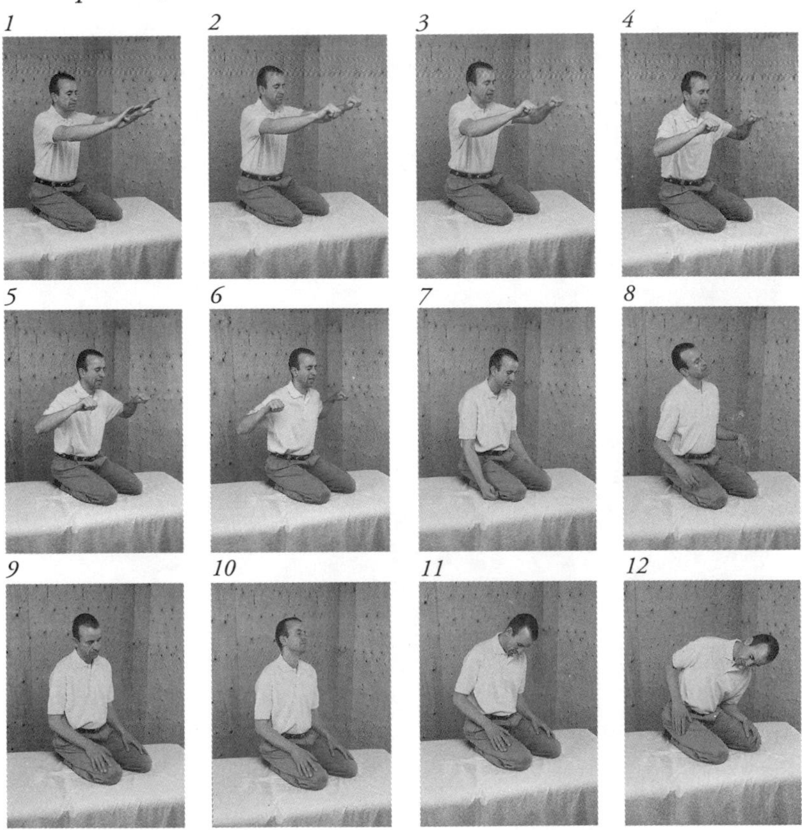

Technique 12—*Reiki Undo:* Reiki Exercise (Self-Practice)

Start with Gassho (s. page 149) and say in your mind, "Reiki exercise start!"

7–12: *Inhale deeply and when you exhale, let go completely. If you are practicing with a partner, touch his or her shoulders from behind and allow your body to move whatever way it wants to (see 13-24 as examples for possible movements.)*

Technique 12—*Reiki Undo:* Reiki Exercise (Practice with a Partner)

13–24: *You sit together in a "train" and say to yourselves: "Reiki Undo start!" Now let the energy move your bodies.*

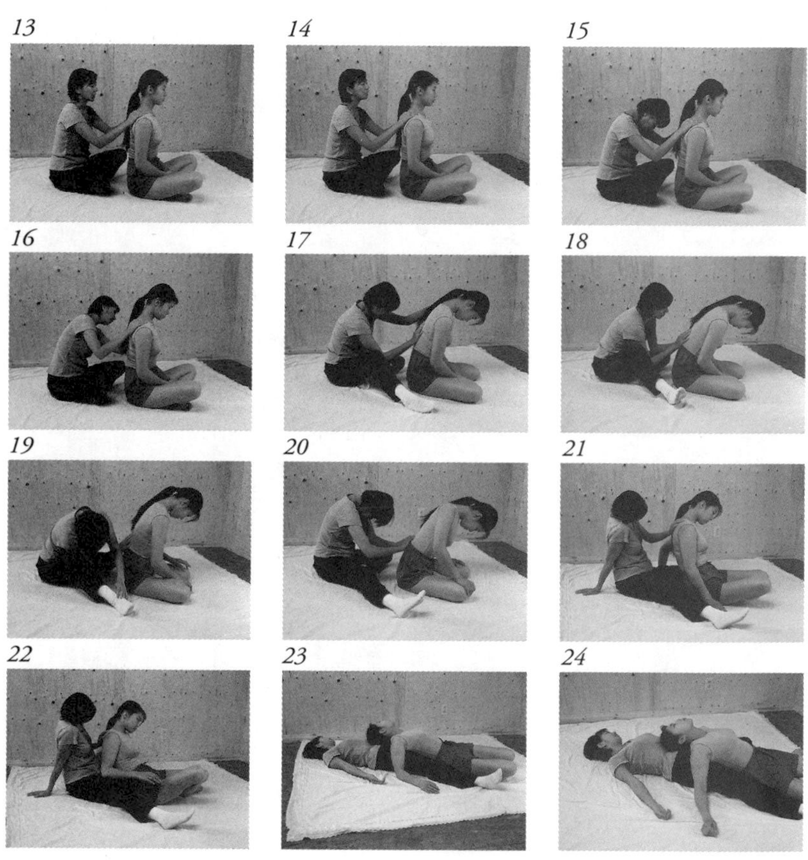
13 *14* *15* *16* *17* *18* *19* *20* *21* *22* *23* *24*

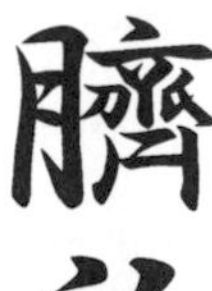
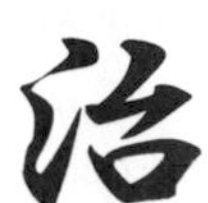
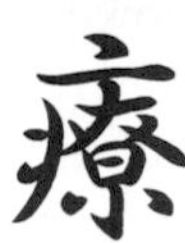

13. *Hesso Chiryo:* The Navel Healing Technique

The Japanese word *hesso* means "navel" and the word *chiryo* means "treatment."

- Place your middle finger in your navel and apply a little pressure until you feel a slight pulse. Do not try to detect the pulse of the abdominal aorta deep inside of your belly. Instead, try to sense the energetic pulse that you can feel when you touch your navel with very gentle pressure. When you have found the pulse, you are ready to start the exercise.
- Let the Reiki energy flow out of your middle finger and into your navel until you feel that your pulse and the energy are in harmony. Practice this for five to ten minutes. The technique can also be used on clients, but please do it very, very gently. Make sure beforehand that clients do not mind having their belly button touched.

Technique 13—*Hesso Chiryo:* Let Energy Flow into the Navel

1: *Place your middle finger in your navel and apply a little pressure until you feel a slight pulse.*
2: *Treating clients*
3: *Self-treatment*

1

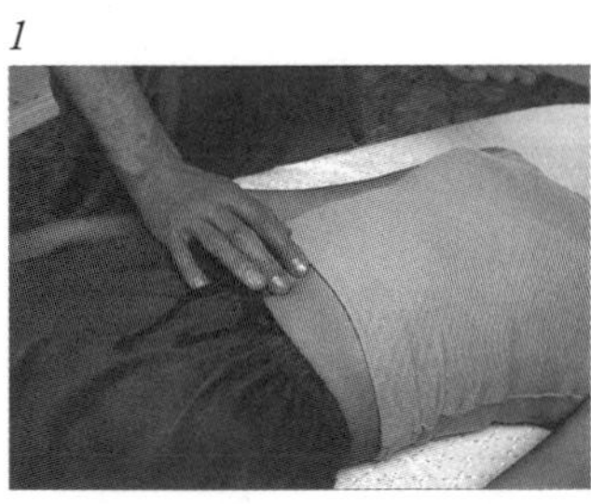

2

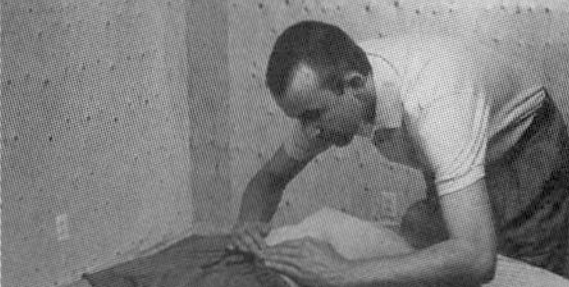

3

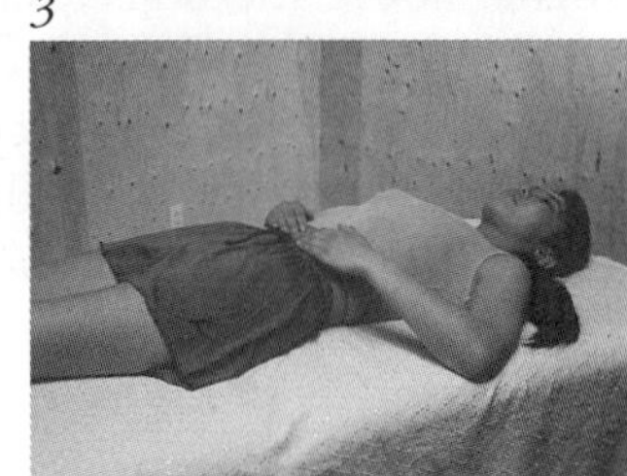

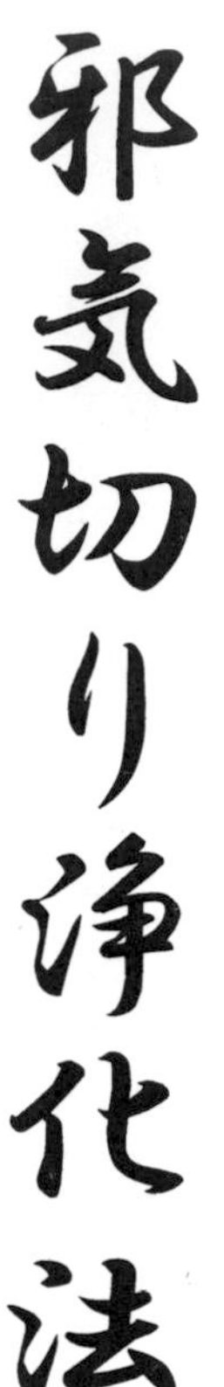

14. *Jacki-Kiri Joka-Ho:* Transforming Negative Energy

The Japanese word *jacki* means negative energy and the word *kiri* (from the verb *kiru*) means "to cut." *Joka-Ho* is a purification technique. It teaches how to cut off negative energy from any object. However, the technique has an important restriction: *Never use it on a living being.* We have other purification techniques available for living beings, like *kenyoku, joshin kokyuu-ho*, and *hanshin koketsu-ho.*

We all know that any object may take on outside energy. Some objects—like crystals, gemstones, and metals—take on energy more readily than others. Many of us have experienced the occasional feeling of "eeeek—what is this?" after either buying something at an antique store or inheriting an item from a relative. We may be feeling the energy of the person who wore or used the object or the energy of the place where the object was kept. If the person was a saint or the place was a holy spot, the object may have become an article of worship. But if the energy attached to the object feels "bad" or uncomfortable, use the technique outlined here. (I put "bad" in quotation marks because energy is never bad. At the most it can be incompatible with us.)

The instructions:

- Hold the object to be purified in your nondominant hand. About 4 inches above the object, cut through the air horizontally with your dominant hand three times. After the third time, stop the movement abruptly. While cutting through the air, stay centered in your tanden and hold your breath. After you have purified the object, give Reiki to it for a few minutes.
- If the object does not fit in your hand, place it on the floor in front of you. If it is too big for you to work on it—like a house, for example—use distant healing.

Technique 14—*Jacki-Kiri Joka-Ho:* Transforming Negative Energy

1–4: *Hold the object to be purified in your nondominant hand. About 2 inches above the object, cut through the air horizontally with your dominant hand three times. After the third time, stop the movement abruptly. While cutting through the air, stay centered in your tanden and hold your breath. After you have purified the object, give Reiki to it for a few minutes.*

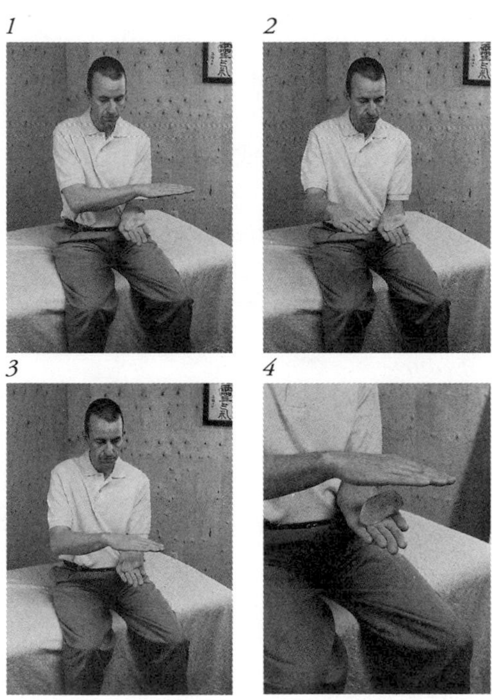

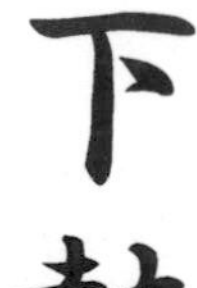

15. *Genetsu-Ho:* The Technique for Bringing Down a Fever

This Japanese word *netsu* means "fever" and the word *ge* means "to bring down."

- Touch the forehead, the temples, the back of the head, the neck, the throat, the crown of the head, the stomach, and the intestines.

This is the standard treatment that Dr. Usui developed for treating any disease of the head, attuning and working on the origin of a disease, and bringing down a fever. Mr. Ogawa suggested leaving the hands on the head positions for about thirty minutes. I usually treat the stomach and intestines for ten to fifteen minutes, allowing my intuition to decide the exact treatment plan in each particular case.

Technique 15—*Genetsu-Ho:* Bringing Down a Fever

Same as techique 16—Byogen Chiryo, see pictures 5-7 (on page 183). This technique can be applied while sitting or lying.

1–7: *Touch the forehead (1), the temples (2), the back of the head (3), the neck (4), the throat (5), the crown of the head (6), the stomach and the intestines (7).*

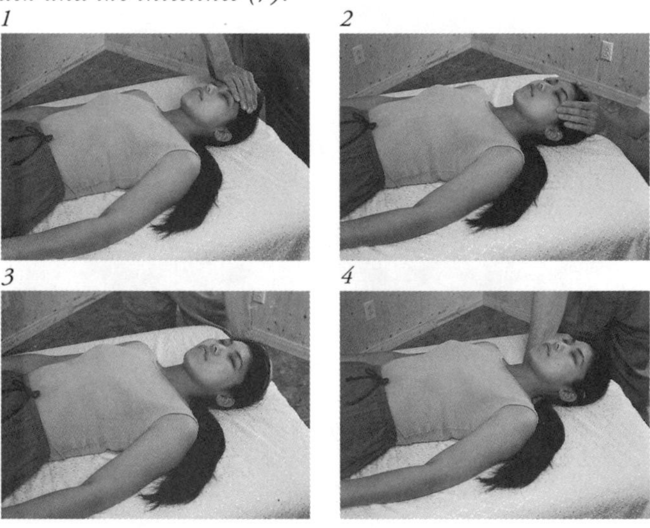

1 *2* *3* *4*

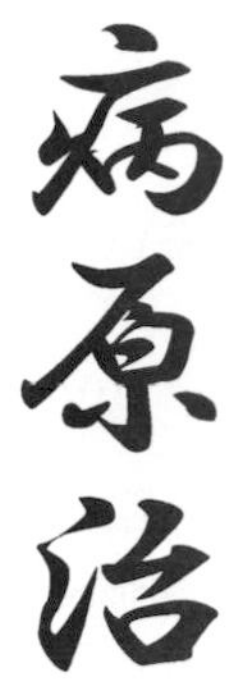

16. *Byogen Chiryo:* Treatment of the Origin of a Disease

The Japanese word *byo* means "disease" and the word *gen* means "origin" or "root."

- The treatment prescribed by Dr. Usui is the same as the *Genetsu-Ho* technique and the treatment of the head.
- Treating the head, stomach, and intestines covers most of the important areas. It is likely you will get a clear picture of your client's physical condition.

We are all aware that what we call a disease is often just a symptom. Treating a symptom will often (but not always) only have a superficial or temporary result. When someone complains of a headache, the actual problem may be located in the spine or be due to dehydration. When we work with the aforementioned *Reiji* technique, (see technique 2 on page 150-152) it is possible to discover the root cause of a disease. Then we should learn to listen to our intuition instead of the symptom description given by the client!

Technique 16—*Byogen Chiryo:* Treatment of the Origin of a Disease

Same as techique 15—Genetsu-Ho, see pictures 1-4 (on page 182). This technique can be applied while sitting or lying.

5

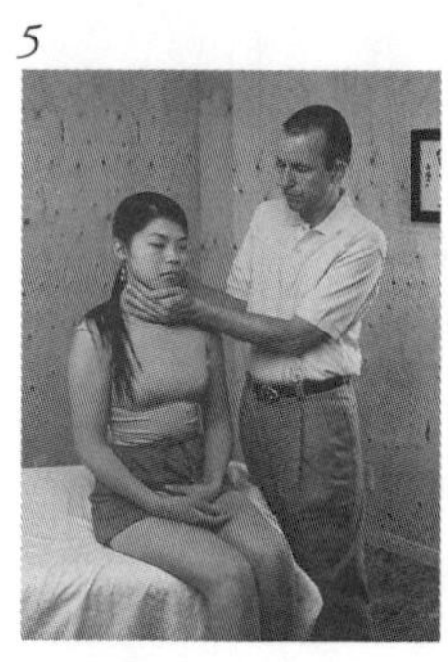

6

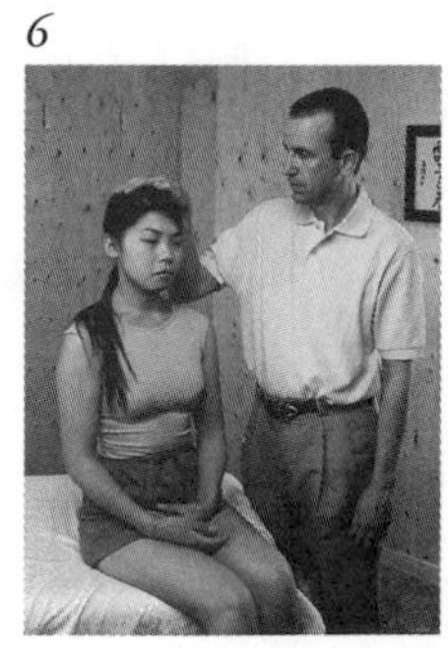

7

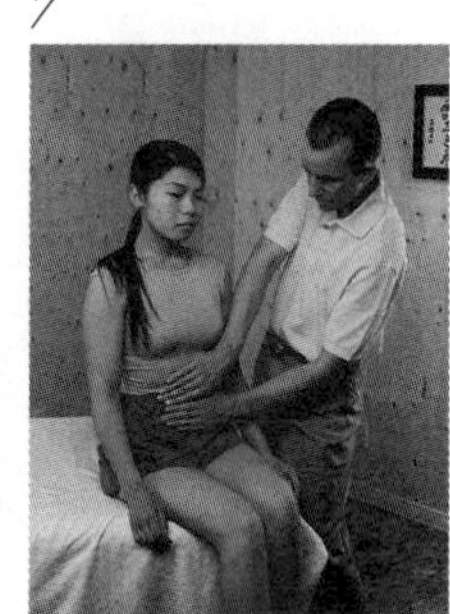

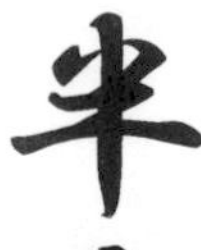

17. *Hanshin Chiryo:* Treatment for Half of the Body

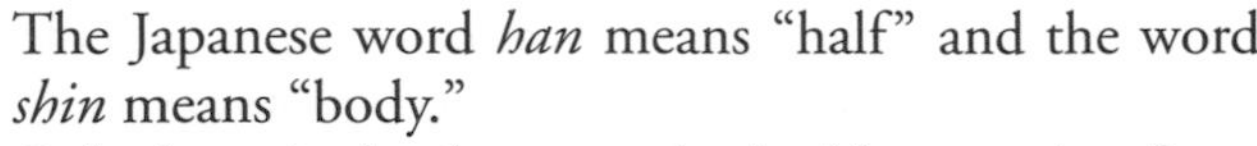

The Japanese word *han* means "half" and the word *shin* means "body."

- Rub the spinal column on both sides, moving from the buttocks to the *medulla oblongata.*

This technique helps a client relax. It is very soothing to have both sides of the spinal column gently rubbed. In Dr. Usui's handbook, the technique is prescribed for disorders of the nerves, as well as disorders of the metabolism and the blood.

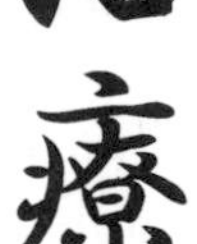

Technique 17—*Hanshin Chiryo*: Treatment for Half of the Body

1–6: *Rub the spinal column on both sides, moving from the buttocks to the medulla oblongata.*

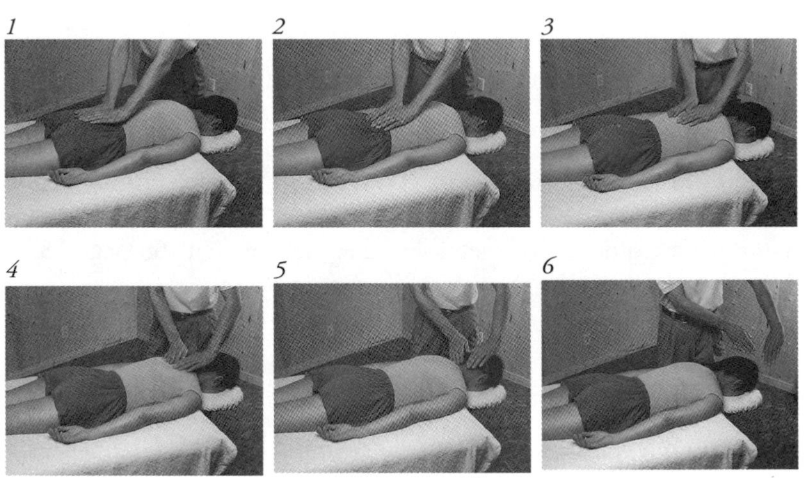

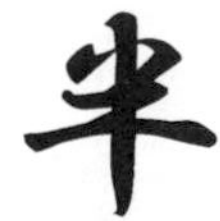

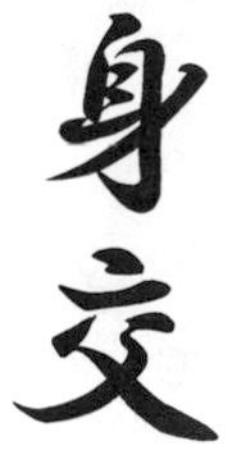

18. *Hanshin Koketsu-Ho:* The Blood-Exchange Technique

As we have seen before, the Japanese word *hanshin* means "half of the body," and *koketsu* can be translated as "cross-blood" or "exchanging, mixing blood." The technique is used to bring a client back down to planet Earth after a treatment. It is also useful when working with mentally disturbed clients.

The instructions:

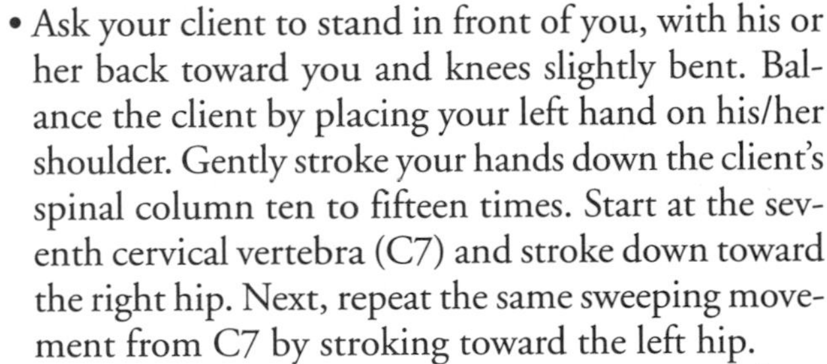

- Ask your client to stand in front of you, with his or her back toward you and knees slightly bent. Balance the client by placing your left hand on his/her shoulder. Gently stroke your hands down the client's spinal column ten to fifteen times. Start at the seventh cervical vertebra (C7) and stroke down toward the right hip. Next, repeat the same sweeping movement from C7 by stroking toward the left hip.
- As you stroke down the spine, hold your breath. After ten to fifteen strokes place your index finger on the left side of the spine and your middle finger on the right side of the spine. Then stroke straight down toward the buttocks. When you reach the point below the fifth lumbar vertebra, apply a little pressure with both fingers and hold it there for a second or two.

Technique 18—*Hanshin Koketsu-Ho:* Blood-Exchange

1–3: *Gently stroke your hands down the his/her spinal column ten to fifteen times. Start at the seventh cervical vertebra (C7) and stroke down toward the right hip. Next, repeat the same sweeping movement from C7 by stroking toward the left hip.*

4–12: *As you stroke down the spine, hold your breath. After ten to fifteen strokes place your index finger on the left side of the spine and your middle finger on the right side of the spine. Then stroke straight down toward the buttocks. When you reach the point below the fifth lumbar vertebra, apply a little pressure with both fingers and hold it there for a second or two.*

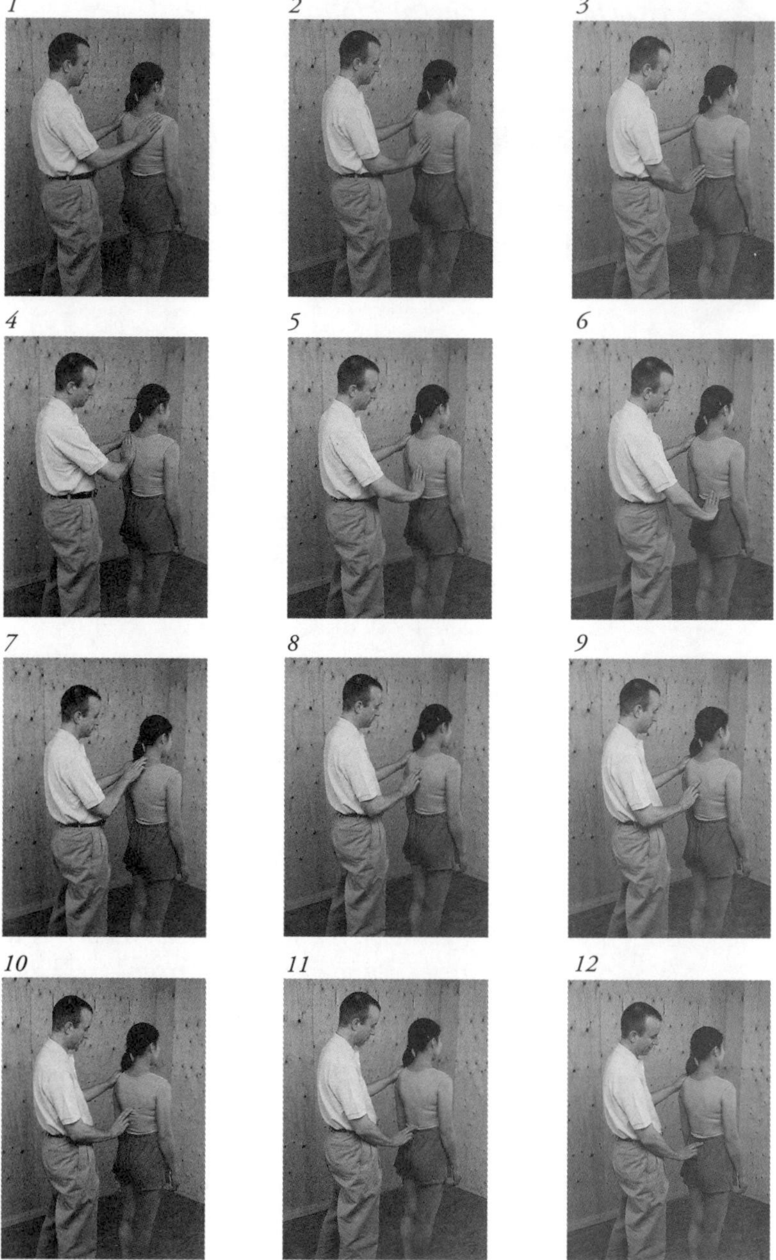
1
2
3
4
5
6
7
8
9
10
11
12

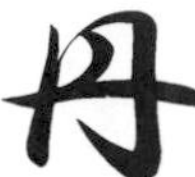

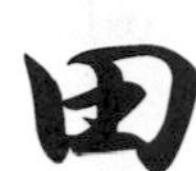

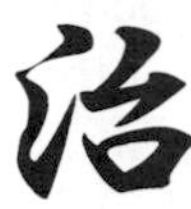

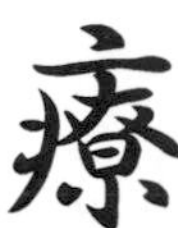

19. *Tanden Chiryo:* Tanden Treatment

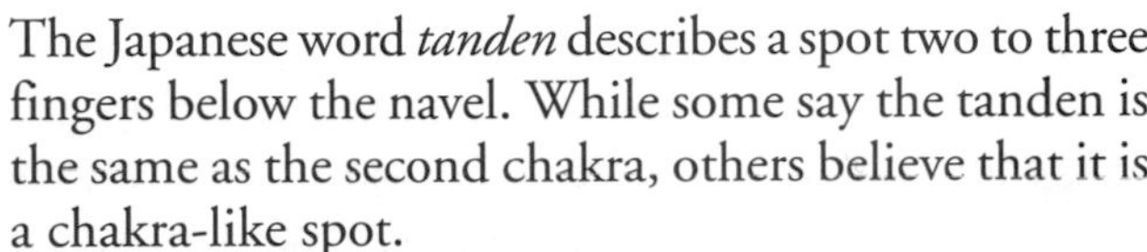
The Japanese word *tanden* describes a spot two to three fingers below the navel. While some say the tanden is the same as the second chakra, others believe that it is a chakra-like spot.

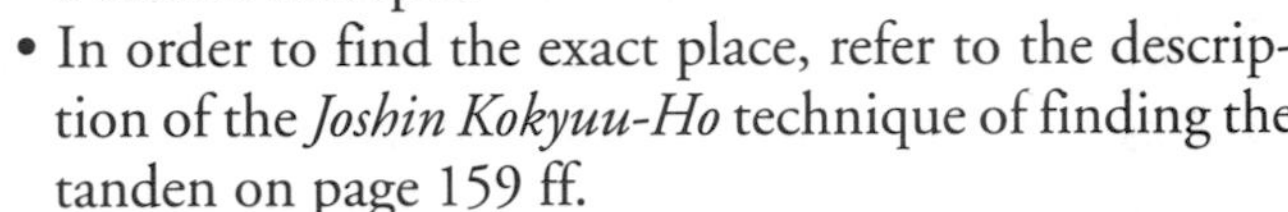
- In order to find the exact place, refer to the description of the *Joshin Kokyuu-Ho* technique of finding the tanden on page 159 ff.
- Once you have found the right spot, place one hand on your tanden and the other on the back of the body behind the tanden. Keep your hands here until they lift off by themselves.

Tanden Chiryo is used as a general power-up technique for yourself or others. It can also strengthen your or your client's willpower.

Technique 19—*Tanden Chiryo:* Tanden Treatment
1–2: *Place one hand on your tanden and the other on the back of the body behind the tanden.*

1

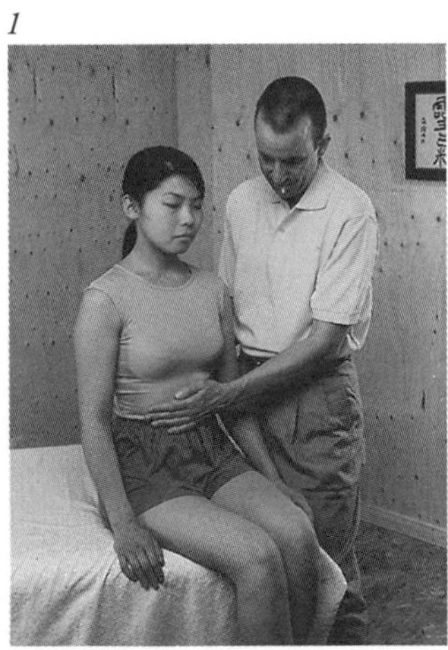

2

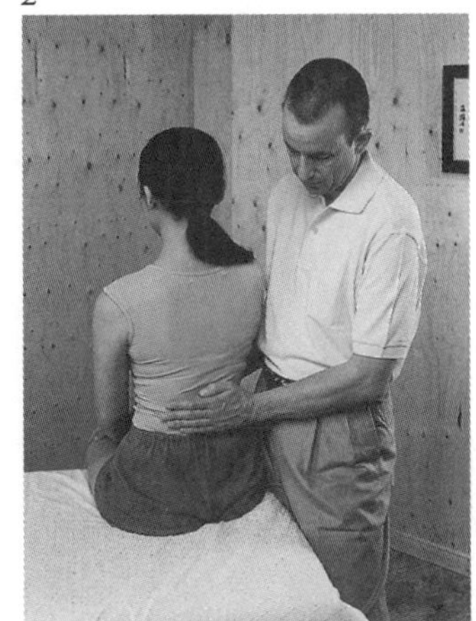

下毒法 20. *Gedoku-Ho:* The Detoxification Technique

The Japanese word *doku* means "poison" or "toxin," and the word ge means "to bring down." The technique is used to detoxify a client or yourself.

- Place one hand on your tanden and the other behind it on the lower back. Leave your hands there for thirteen minutes while simultaneously imagining all the toxins leaving the body of the Reiki receiver. It helps to ask the recipient to imagine the same.

I personally imagine the toxins leaving the recipient through the feet, going down into the ground. Don't worry about poisoning the Earth. The Earth easily turns the energies into life-giving nutrients.

This technique helps to counteract the side effects of medicines.

Technique 20—*Gedoku-Ho:* Detoxification

1–2: *Place one hand on your tanden and the other behind it on the lower back. Leave your hands there for thirteen minutes while simultaneously imagining all the toxins leaving the body of the Reiki receiver.*

1

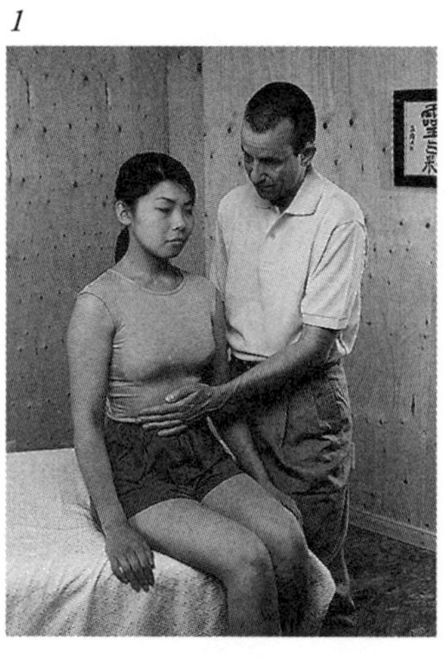

2

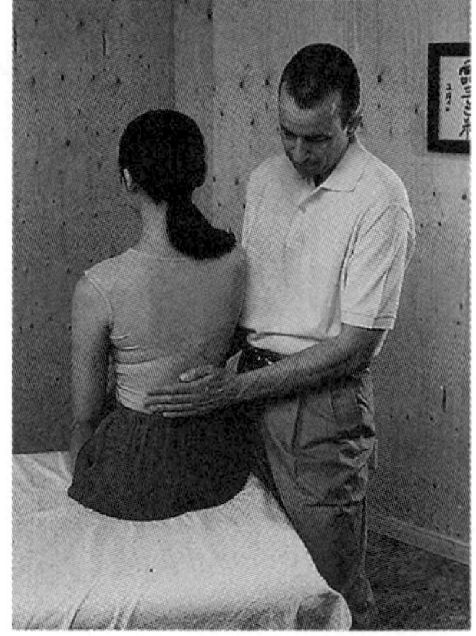

A Little Food for Thought

One more thought at the end of the chapter: Techniques are fingers pointing to the moon. They are tools and not to be confused with the "real thing." YOU are the real thing. YOU are the moon and not the finger pointing to it. Beyond thoughts and emotions, body and soul, good and bad, health and disease, Reiki energy, all your concepts, your dreams, and aspirations, you are it!

Always ask yourself who is doing the experiencing. At the end of the day, the only question that remains is, "Who Am I, Who Am I, Who Am I?" When that question is answered, all suffering comes to an end.

CHAPTER 19

Healing Techniques According to Dr. Chujiro Hayashi*

—translation of the Japanese original by Midori Egi
© 1998 by William Lee Rand—

Hayashi Reiki Institute, American Branch

(This printed copy is a substitute for the original handwritten text.)

This hand-position guide for Reiki treatments is a translation of the manual used by Dr. Hayashi that he gave to his students. It lists various illnesses and conditions and indicates which hand positions to use to treat them.

Healing Techniques

Chapter 1:
HEAD

1. Head: ***Brain diseases, headache***
1. front of jaw, 2. temples, 3. back of the head and back of the neck, 4. top of the head [note: With any disease you can include head treatment as a part of the disease treatment. In the case of a headache, you should treat very thoroughly the place on the head that is aching.]

* Please notice that this chapter is a reproduction of an old original Japanese text, and is to be used exclusively for explanatory purposes. (This information is intended for interested readers and educational purposes only. The readers are not to diagnose or treat on illness by themselves. For diagnosis and treatment of any illness we recommend visiting a medical professional.)

2. Eyes: ***All kinds of eye diseases: conjunctivitis, trachoma, leucoma, nearsightedness, trichiasis, ptosis, cataract, glaucoma, etc.***
1. eye balls, 2. inside corners of eyes, 3. outside corners of eyes, 4. back of the head [note: Even though one eye has a problem, you treat both eyes. You also treat the kidneys, liver, womb, and ovaries.]

3. Ears: ***All kinds of ear diseases, tympanitis, external otitis, ringing ear, hard of hearing, etc.***
1, auditory canal, 2. depression just below the ears, 3. high bone behind the ears, 4. back of the head [note: Even though one ear has a problem, you treat both ears. In the case of diseases that follow colds, such as tympanitis and parotitis, you must treat bronchi and hilar lymph. Also pay attention to the kidneys, womb, and ovaries.]

4. Teeth
In the case of a toothache, treat from the outside at the root of the tooth.

5. Oral cavity
Shut the mouth, and then treat the lips by holding the palms on them [note: see *Diseases of Digestive Organs*]

6. Tongue
1. Press on or pinch the diseased part of the tongue. 2. Treat the root of the tongue from outside the mouth. [note: If you find this technique difficult, then press both arches of the feet forward.]

Chapter 2: DISEASES OF DIGESTIVE ORGANS

1. Stomatitis
1. mouth, 2. esophagus, 3. stomach, 4. intestines, 5. liver

2. Thrush
1. mouth, 2. tongue, 3. esophagus, 4. stomach, 4. intestines, 6. liver, 7. heart, 8. kidneys [note: To heal the tongue, treat the arches of the feet.]

3. Saliva
1. mouth, 2. root of the tongue, 3. stomach, 4. intestines, 5. head

4. Esophagus diseases: ***Stricture of the esophagus, dilation of the esophagus, esophagitis***
1. esophagus, 2. cardia (solar plexus), 3. stomach, 4. intestines, 5. liver, 6. pancreas, 7. kidneys, 8. blood exchange* [note: In the case of esophagus cancer, the prognosis is most likely not very good.]

5. Stomach diseases: ***Acute and chronic gastritis, gastric atony, gastric dilation, gastric ulcer, stomach cancer, gastroptosis, neurologic stomach ache, neurologic dyspepsia,*** **gastrospasm**
1. stomach, 2. liver, 3. pancreas, 4. intestines, 5. kidneys, 6. spinal cord, 7. blood exchange [note: If the condition of the cancer is obvious, the prognosis is most likely not very good.]

6. Intestinal diseases: ***Intestinal catarrh, constipation, appendicitis, vermiform process, ileus, invagination, intestinal volvulus, intestinal bleeding, diarrhea***
1. stomach, 2. intestines, 3. liver, 4. pancreas, 5. kidneys, 6. heart, 7. blood exchange, 8. lumbar vertebrae, 9. sacrum

7. Liver diseases: ***Liver congestion, hyperemia, abscess, sclerosis, hypertrophy, atrophy, jaundice, gallstone, etc.***
1. liver, 2. pancreas, 3. stomach, 4. intestines, 5. heart, 6. kidneys, 7. blood exchange [note: A few days after the treatment, gallstones will break into pieces by themselves and will be eliminated from the body. In the case of liver cancer, prognosis is most likely not very good.]

8. Pancreatic diseases: ***Liver cyst, ptosis, hypertrophy, etc.***
1. pancreas, 2. liver, 3. stomach, 4. intestines, 5. heart, 6. kidneys, 7. blood exchange [note: In the case of pancreatic cancer, prognosis is most likely not very good.]

---

* Blood exchange: This technique will be mentioned very often in the following pages. It will be explained on page 202.

9. Peritoneum diseases
1. liver, 2. pancreas, 3. stomach, 4. intestines, 5. peritoneum area, 6. bladder, 7. heart, 8. kidneys, 9. blood exchange [note: In the case of tuberculosis diseases, treat the lung area.]

10. Anal diseases: ***Hemorrhoid, inflammation of anus area, open sores of anus area, bleeding piles, anal fistula, prolapse of the anus***
1. the affected part of anus, 2. coccyges, 3. stomach, 4. intestines [note: In the case of anal fistula, do the same treatment as intestinal and pulmonary tuberculosis.]

Chapter 3: RESPIRATORY DISEASES

1. Nasal diseases: ***Acute and chronic nasal catarrh, hypertrophic and atrophic nasal catarrh***
1. nose, 2. throat, 3. bronchi

2. Maxillary empyema
1. nose, 2. depression of upper and front jaw, 3. chest, 4. throat, 5. kidneys, 6. stomach, 7. intestines, 8. blood exchange

3. Nosebleed (epistaxis)
1. nasal bones, 2. back of the head [note: If menstruation is late and nosebleed occurs, treat the womb and ovaries.]

4. Sore throat and tonsillitis
1. throat, 2. tonsil, 3. bronchi, 4. kidneys, 5. lungs, 6. stomach, 7. intestines, 8. head [note: In the case of tonsillitis, treat the kidneys well.]

5. Tracheitis and bronchitis
1. tracheas and bronchi, 2. lungs, 3. stomach, 4. intestines, 5. heart, 6. kidneys, 7. head

6. Pneumonia: ***Catarrhalcroupous***
1.lungs, 2. bronchi, 3. heart, 4. liver, 5. pancreas, 6. stomach, 7. intestines, 8. kidneys, 9. blood exchange

7. Asthma: ***Chronic and acute asthma***
1. bronchi, 2. lungs, 3. liver, 4. pancreas, 5. diaphragm, 6. stomach, 7. intestines, 8. kidneys, 9. head, 10. nose,11. heart [note: In the case of an acute attack, you may let your patient sit up and treat them in this position.]

8. Lung diseases: ***Pulmonary edema, abscess, pulmonary tuberculosis, emphysema of lungs***
1. lung area, 2. heart, 3. liver, 4. pancreas, 5. stomach, 6. intestines, 7. bladder, 8. kidneys, 9. spinal cord, 10. head [note: In the case of women, regardless of their age, always treat the womb and ovaries. Doing blood exchange is effective, but do not do it with very weak and very sick patients.]

9. Pleura diseases: ***Both dry and moist***
1. chest area in general, 2. heart, 3. liver, 4. pancreas, 5. stomach, 6. intestines, 7. kidneys, 8. blood exchange

Chapter 4: CARDIOVASCULAR DISEASES

1. Heart diseases: ***Endocarditis, heart valve diseases, various symptoms of pericardium, various symptoms of the heart itself, palpitation, angina pectoris, etc.***
1. heart, 2. liver, 3. stomach, 4. intestines, 5. pancreas, 6. kidneys, 7. spinal cord, 8. blood exchange

2. Arteriosclerosis: ***Aneurysm, cardiac asthma, etc.***
1. same as treating heart problems, 2. bronchi and chest area

Chapter 5:
URINARY ORGAN DISEASES:

1. Kidney diseases: ***Kidney congestion, anemia, atrophy, sclerosis, hypertrophy, abscess, wandering kidney, pyelitis, kidney stone, uremia, filariasis***
1. kidneys, 2. liver, 3. pancreas, 4. heart, 5. stomach, 6. intestines 7. bladder, 8. head, 9. blood exchange

2. Cystitis: ***Urinary retention, uremia, urgency, pain when urinating***
1. kidneys, 2. bladder, 3. urethra, 4. prostate gland, 5. wombs, 6. same as treating kidney diseases

3. Enuvesis
1. bladder, 2. intestines, 3. stomach, 4. kidneys, 5. spinal cord, 6. head, 7. blood exchange

Chapter 6:
NEUROLOGICAL DISEASES

1. Cerebral anemia, cerebral hyperemia
1. head, 2. heart

2. Hysteria
1. womb, 2. ovaries, 3. stomach, 4. intestines, 5. liver, 6. kidneys, 7. head, 8. eyes, 9. blood exchange

3. Nervous breakdown, insomnia
1. stomach, 2. intestines, 3. liver, 4. pancreas, 5. kidneys, 6. eyes, 7. head, 8. blood exchange [note: Be careful with maxillary empyema.]

4. Meningitis

1. head, mainly back of the head and back of the neck [note: Mainly treat the head in order to heal the cause of the disease, such as the nose, forehead, and inflammation of the head; also in order to heal remote organs' diseases, such as gastiritis and pneumonia caused by erysipelas. Same for tuberculous.]

5. Epidemic cerebrospinal meningitis

1. spinal cord 2. back of the head and back of the neck 3. heart, 4. stomach, 5. intestines, 6. liver, 7. kidneys, 8. bladder [note: Mainly treat the spinal cord, back of the head, and back of the neck.]

6. Myelitis

1. spinal cord in general, 2. stomach, 3. intestines, 4. liver, 5. bladder, 6. kidneys, 7. head, 8. blood exchange

7. Cerebral hemorrhage, intracerebral bleeding, cerebral thrombosis, etc. ,

1. head, 2. heart, 3. kidneys, 4. stomach, 5. intestines, 6. liver, 7. spinal cord, 8. paralyzed area

8. Polio

1. spinal cord, 2. stomach, 3. intestines, 4. kidneys, 5. sacrum, 6. paralyzed area, 7. head, 8. blood exchange

9. Neuralgia, palsy, neural spasticity, migraine

1. affected area, 2. liver, 3. pancreas, 4. stomach, 5. intestines, 6. kidneys, 7. head, 8. spinal cord, 9. blood exchange [note: Pay attention to the womb and ovaries.]

10. Beriberi

1. stomach, 2. intestines, 3. heart, 4. liver, 5. pancreas, 6. kidneys, 7. paralyzed or edematous area 8. blood exchange

11. Graves' disease

1. womb, 2. ovaries, 3. stomach, 4. intestines, 5. liver, 6. pancreas, 7. heart, 8. thyroid, 9. eyes, 10. kidneys, 11. spinal cord 12. blood exchange

12. Epilepsy
1. liver, 2. pancreas, 3. head, 4. stomach, 5. intestines, 6. kidneys, 7. spinal cord, 8. blood exchange

13. Convulsion
1. liver, 2. stomach, 3. intestines, 4. kidneys, 5. spinal cord, 6. shoulders, 7. arms, 8. elbow joint area, 9. wrist, 10. head

14. Chorea
1. liver, 2. stomach, 3. intestines, 4. kidneys, 5. spinal cord, 6. spastic area at the legs and arms, 7. head, 8. blood exchange

15. Sea sick
1. stomach, 2. solar plexus, 3. head

16. Food poisoning
1. stomach, 2. solar plexus, 3. liver, 4. pancreas, 5. intestines, 6. heart, 7. kidneys, 8. head, 9. blood exchange

Chapter 7:
INFECTIOUS DISEASES

1. Typhoid, paratyphy
1. liver,, 2. pancreas (spleen), 3. stomach, 4. intestines, 5. heart, 6. kidneys, 7. spinal cord, 8. head,

2. Dysentery: ***Cholera, children's dysentery and others***
1. stomach,, 2. intestines, 3. liver, 4. pancreas, 5. kidneys, 6. heart, 7. head, 8. blood exchange

3. Measles
1. throat, 2. trachea, 3. bronchi, 4. stomach, 5. intestines, 6. heart 7. kidneys, 8. spinal cord, 9. head

4. Scarlet fever
1. throat, 2. chest, 3. kidneys, 4. stomach, 5. intestines, 6. bladder, 7. head, 8. blood exchange

5. Varicella

1. stomach, 2. intestines, 3. kidneys, 4. blood exchange, 5. affected area, 6. head

6. Influenza

1. nose, 2. throat,, 3. trachea,, 4. bronchi,, 5. lungs 6. liver, 7. pancreas, 8. stomach, 9. intestines, 10. kidneys, 11. head, 12. blood exchange

7. Whooping cough

1. nose, 2. throat, 3. bronchi, 4. apex of the lungs, 5. stomach, 6. intestines, 7. kidneys, 8. blood exchange

8. Diphtheria

1. throat, 2. trachea, 3. nose, 4. lungs, 5. heart, 6. liver, 7. stomach, 8. intestines, 9. kidneys, 10. blood exchange

9. Malaria

1. pancreas (spleen), 2. liver, 3. heart, 4. stomach, 5. intestines, 6. kidneys, 7. spinal cord, 8. blood exchange

10. Tetanus

1. jawbone, 2. back of head, 3. throat, 4. lungs, 5. affected area, 6. stomach, 7. intestines, 8. kidneys, 9. spinal cord [note: In the case of puerperal tetanus, treat the womb. In the case of primary child, treat the navel.]

11. Articular rheumatism, muscular rheumatism

1. affected area, 2. heart, 3. chest,4. liver, 5. pancreas, 6. stomach, 7. intestines, 8. kidneys, 9. spinal cord 10. head,

12. Rabies

1. affected area, 2. heart, 3. liver, 4. kidneys, 5. stomach, 6. intestines, 7. spinal cord, 8. throat, 9. head, 10. blood exchange

Chapter 8:
WHOLE BODY DISEASES

1. Anemia, leukemia, scorbutus
1. heart, 2. liver, 3. pancreas, 4. stomach, 5. intestines, 6. kidneys, 7. spinal cord, 8. blood exchange

2. Diabetes
1. liver, 2. pancreas, 3. heart, 4. stomach, 5. intestines, 6. bladder, 7. kidneys, 8. head, 9. spinal cord, 10. blood exchange

3. Dermatological diseases
1. stomach, 2. intestines, 3. liver, 4. kidneys, 5. affected area, 6. blood exchange

4. Obesity (adiposis)
The same as diabetes.

5. Scrofula
1. affected area, 2. stomach, 3. intestines, 4. liver, 5. heart, 6. chest, 7. kidneys, 8. spinal cord, 9. blood exchange

Chapter 9:
OTHER DISEASES

1. Infantile convulsion
1. heart, 2. head, 3. stomach, 4. intestines

2. Wrong position of fetus
1. womb

3. Pregnancy
1. If you treat the womb continually, the growth of fetus is healthy.

4. Delivery

1. Sacrum 2. lumbar spine [note: If you treat these areas, after twelve labor pains the baby will be born very easily. If you keep on treating these areas after the birth of the baby, the afterbirth will be easy as well.]

5. Death of fetus

1. If you treat the womb, the dead fetus will naturally come out on the same day or the next day.

6. Cessation of mother's milk

If you treat around the breast and mammary gland, the mother will soon start having milk.

7. Morning sickness

1. womb, 2. stomach, 3. solar plexus, 4. intestines, 5. kidneys, 6. head, 7. spinal cord

8. Erysipelas

1. affected area, 2. stomach, 3. intestines, 4. liver, 5. heart, 6. kidneys, 7. spinal cord, 8. blood exchange

9. Hyperhidrosis

1. kidneys, 2. affected area, 3. blood exchange

10. Burn

Put one hand one or two inches away from the affected area. When the pain is gone, put the hand on this area.

11. Cut by a sword

Treat as you press the cut with a thumb or a palm to prevent bleeding.

12. Unconsciousness by falling, an electric shock. etc.

1. *katsu**, 2. heart, 3. head

---

* *Katsu*: A technique to revive those who have lost consciousness. It will not be explained in detail here.

13. Drowning
1. let the patient throw up water, 2. *katsu**, 3. heart, 4. head

14. Menopause, period pains
1. womb, 2. ovaries, 3. cranium

15. Hiccup
1. diaphragm, 2. liver, 3. pancreas, 4. kidneys, 5. stomach, 6. intestines, 7. spinal cord, 8. head

16. Stuttering
1. throat, 2. head, 3. singing practice

Practice song number 1:
Mukou no Koike ni "Dojo" ga sanbiki nyoro-nyoro to. (There are three loaches wiggling in the pond over there.)

Practice song number 2:
2. Oya ga Kahyo nara ko ga Kahyo. Ko-Kahyo ni Mago-Kahyo. (The parent is Kahyo, his child is Kahyo. Son, Kahyo and grandson, Kahyo.) [note: Those who can sing songs can be healed.]

17. Pain at the tip of fingers
1. affected area

18. Vomiting
1. stomach, 2. solar plexus, 3. liver, 4. spinal cord at the back of stomach,5. head, 6. kidneys

19. Splinter
1. affected area [note: When the pain leaves, the splinter comes back. You pull the splinter out at this moment.]

20. Gonorrhea,
1. urethra, 2. Hui-Yin, 3. bladder, 4. womb [note: If it is orchitis, apply your hand lightly on the testicles.]

21. Spasm of pain, stomach cramps

1. stomach, 2. on the back at the stomach, 3. liver, 4. kidneys, 5. intestines, 6. head

22. Hernia

As you touch the affected area lightly, it will contract by itself. Treat stomach and intestines.

Explanatory Notes:

Blood Exchange, *Ketsueki-Kokan.* It is a technique to get rid of dirty blood, or dirty substances from the body. You stroke along the back bone of the patient from neck downward. *[Note from William Lee Rand:* this technique is to release negative energy from the aura of the patient.]

CHAPTER 20

The Systematic Whole Body Treatment with Reiki

—by Walter Lübeck—

In the First Degree of the Usui System of Natural Healing, the "major remedy" is the systematic whole body treatment. In this form of treatment, a person who has been initiated into the Reiki methods lays hands on his or her own body or someone else's body according to a specific system. Every three to five minutes, the positions are changed. If the course of the whole body treatment has been designed in a meaningful way, the beneficial effects of the Reiki transmission mutually support each other from every position. This creates synergy effects and a substantially better and deeper-reaching treatment results than we would actually presume at first glance considering the relatively short treatment period for each position.

Introduction

Now there are many different forms of whole body treatment with Reiki and this diversity can be quite confusing. Which one is the right one? Which one helps the most? There certainly isn't just *one* optimal form of whole body treatment but a number of meaningful approaches. In any case, it is better to give Reiki—even if the order of the positions does not mutually support the effect in an optimal manner—than not applying the universal life energy at all.

Yet, with a whole body treatment that has been designed with the appropriate expertise, you can work more effectively in every way than by just laying the hands on the various areas of the body. There is naturally also the possibility of using Reiki intuitively. But, in most cases, this must first be learned well. Feeling is not always the same as intuition. Moreover, the systematic whole body treatment is also the basis for an intuitive treatment approach. Apart from this factor, the whole body treatment is also a wonderful method for beginners (and others) to train their sensitivity and subtle perception on various levels and learn to open up to other people with all of their senses in a heart-felt way.

In order to provide an orientation that can easily be practiced, this chapter precisely describes the implementation and effects of each position for the form of whole body treatment that I have optimized in years of experience. On the one hand, this can be helpful if you want to learn a well-functioning treatment method for practically any case; on the other hand, a great deal can be learned about the subtle energy system of human beings and psychosomatic correlations through the commentaries on the positions. These sections extensively explain how a treatment with Reiki can fundamentally be enriched through the synergy effects. On this basis, those who have adequate practical experience can begin to develop their own method of whole body treatment or an abridged form of it for special purposes.[27]

The best approach is to first read this chapter from beginning to end. Then begin practicing the whole body treatment. Pay attention to the various sensations in your hands during each of the positions. Notice how the feeling of your body changes and how your client behaves. After the treatment, take notes on your perceptions during each position and read the commentaries on the individual hand positions again. Consider the various correlations and talk to your clients about it. This is how I learned most quickly and it has also helped many Reiki students find the best approach to the universal life energy. You may also find it helpful.

General Information on the Reiki Whole Body Treatment

The whole body treatment is, as already explained above, the major remedy of the Reiki method. It can be used at any time for the maintenance or optimization of your physical or psychic well-being—or just because it is so wonderful to pamper yourself with it.

If you are not ill, the whole body treatment will help you to be fit and make the best out of your possibilities. Mikao Usui, the founder of the Reiki method, said that the most fascinating effect of Reiki for him was that it helps people develop their slumbering talents, find their path to the light, and become more alive. He considered the health benefits as secondary to this aim. Usui saw Reiki as a spiritual path. Why shouldn't Reiki be used on a regular basis, even without the necessity of an illness? It's best to indulge in it regularly, allowing Reiki to be absorbed for at least three minutes in each position. And more than that doesn't hurt.

If you give yourself a whole body treatment one to three times a week, you will soon notice a steady increase in

- vitality
- creativity
- sensitivity and intuition
- strength
- endurance
- inner peace and
- joy in life.

Many people who use Reiki report that the tendency toward illnesses such as colds, digestive disorders, or headaches is distinctly reduced and often is even cured by regular applications of Reiki. So remember:

Reiki once a day keeps the doctor away!

There is naturally a difference between whether you treat yourself or let someone else pamper you with a whole body treatment. In the first case, you must be active yourself and assume responsibility; in the second case, you don't need to worry about anything. You can simply relax and enjoy the blessings of the universal life energy. However, the positions (treated zones of the body) are always the same for both self-treatment and giving treatments to others. Because of anatomical reasons, you will naturally place the hands differently on your own body—the person giving the treatment should also be comfortable while doing so.

Within the scope of the Reiki method, it isn't important which hand you put where, the direction in which the fingers point, and the like since Reiki is a non-polar energy form. However, treatment is always given with the palm of the hand because this is where the secondary chakras responsible for transmitting Reiki are located. Treatment can be given with body contact or at a short distance from the body. One to a maximum of two handbreadths distance from the surface of the body are usually appropriate in this technique. In the latter case, it can be useful to apply the cloud-hands technique; to do this, move your hands slightly back and forth as if they were dancing in the wind. Let your body be in control. There usually isn't a very big difference between whether treatment is done with contact or without it. In case of doubt, you can simply try it out for yourself. Always hold your hands in a way that is comfortable for you.

The Proper Preparation for a Whole Body Treatment

Neither the client nor the treatment-giver should be under the influence of intoxicating drugs during a Reiki whole body treatment. This also includes alcohol, strong coffee, and tobacco products. The consumption of drugs reduces the body's ability to resonate and therefore the possibility of stimulating its self-healing powers through Reiki. In addition, intoxicating drugs also strain the detoxification organs in a purely biochemical way. As a result, the breaking down and elimination of toxins and waste materials stored in the body is drastically reduced. The consumption of alcohol should therefore stop at least eight hours before the Reiki session so that the effect of the treatment is not diminished. According to sensitivity and the amount consumed, a time period of about 30 to 90 minutes before the treatment should be adequate for coffee, black tea, and cigarettes. *Please observe*: This in no way means that Reiki will not be effective or that it will cause damage if this advice isn't taken to heart.

If the person giving the treatment is a smoker, he or she should wear thin gloves (made of latex, for example) that do not allow the smell to come through when treating the client's head and throat area. Since the smell of tobacco can be clearly detected on the hands even hours after the last cigarette, this is otherwise quite unpleasant for non-smokers.

The room should be calm and have a pleasant temperature. Meditation music, which is abundantly available today, usually fits in well with the atmosphere of a Reiki session. The client should have a word in the selection of the music since it is ultimately *his* or *her* hour. Many treatment-givers dispense with music in order to concentrate better on the situation. There are no objections to this approach either, which I frequently use. However, calm and meditative music can help some people let go more easily, inwardly distance themselves from everyday life, and better open up to the gentle, healing touch of Reiki. In case of doubt, I think that the needs of the person receiving Reiki have priority.

Don't use too much incense, strictly making sure that you use natural products. In any case, talk to your client about whether or not to use incense or a fragrance lamp, including which fragrances to use. *Caution:* Some people have allergic reactions to incense and fragrance oils!

Before giving treatment, wash your hands, remove quartz-crystal watches, jewelry (especially closed metal circles such as rings and chains), and loosen tight clothing and belts. *The client* should also remove quartz-crystal watches, jewelry (especially closed metal circles such as rings and chains), loosen tight clothing and belts, and visit the toilet beforehand.

Beginning the Reiki Whole Body Treatment

Attune yourself to the treatment situation, fold your hands in front of your heart, and ask permission to be a channel for Reiki. Ask for healing on all levels for your client and bow to him or her. While bowing, raise your hands to your forehead and lower them back down to your heart when standing up again.

Now smooth out the client's aura in the following manner: with the palm facing the client's body along the center line consciously move one hand *at least* three times at a slow and even pace at the height of about one to two handbreadths, starting at the top of the head down to beyond the tips of the toes. Be sure to keep your hand outside the client's energy field with the palms turned away from him or her when bringing them back up to the top. While doing this, keep your other hand on your hara*. You can find the hara about two fingers below your navel. If you are treating yourself, you can naturally smooth out your aura as well, but you don't need to maintain the contact with your hara. Instead of smoothing the aura, you can take a shower—the first thirty seconds at body temperature, then warm water up to 43° C (109° F) warm or cold water is suitable. For an optimum effect, shower your head as well.

The actual whole body treatment actually begins after this preparation process. Be sure you hold all of your fingers together, including your thumbs. This allows you to give Reiki more intensively. It naturally also flows when you keep the fingers apart, but at a weaker intensity.

* The hara is the energetic center of the human being. It is the point of perfect balance, the true spiritual essence of a being. If you open up to your hara, you will become calm, powerful, and your intuition will function better. This also promotes the here-and-now orientation of the conscious mind.

The 17 Positions of the Reiki Whole Body Treatment

The Head Positions

1. Place the hands to the right and left of the nose, from the forehead to the eyes and the level of the mouth.
2. Your hands should cover the temples, with the fingertips reaching at least to the cheekbones. If you are treating yourself, place the hands so that they completely cover the cheekbones and the temples.
3. Cover the ears with the hands.
4. Place the hands on the back of the head, and be sure to cover the medulla oblongata at the center of the back of the head.
5. Let the hands cover the throat. Do not have any body contact here—in order to avoid fear (sense of strangulation)! As an alternative, you can also place one hand on the back of the neck and the other on the front.

The Trunk Positions

6. Let one hand cover the lower ribs on the right side, extending to the center of the body and the lower edge of the ribs. Place the other hand directly beneath it.
7. Reverse this position on the left side, with one hand covering the lower ribs on the left side and extending to the center of the body and the lower edge of the ribs. Place the other hand directly beneath it.
8. Place one hand above and the other below the navel. The distance between the hands should be about two to three fingers. Reiki radiates quite intensively about two fingers around the hands. Consequently, this distance can be employed to provide a larger area with Reiki by using just this one position.
9. Horizontally place one hand directly below the throat on the thymus gland at the center line of the body and the other vertically on the heart area so that a T-shape is created. When treating yourself, it is more comfortable to place both hands horizontally beneath each other: one hand on the thymus gland and the other about two to three fingers under it, above the heart and bronchial tubes.

10. Beginning with the somewhat protruding pelvic bones to the left and right on the upper pelvic area, place your hands so that they reach the beginning of the pubic bone, forming a type of "V."

The Back Positions

11. Place the hands horizontally between the upper side of the shoulder and the shoulder blades to the right and left of the spinal column. When giving yourself a treatment, it is more comfortable to first give Reiki to one side and then the other. The hand giving the treatment should be very relaxed. Support its elbow with the other hand to hold it in position. If this isn't possible, treat the back from the front at the same height. In this case, be sure to give about 10 minutes of Reiki instead of 3 minutes.
12. Let your hands horizontally cover the shoulder blades. When giving yourself the treatment, it is more comfortable to first give Reiki to one side and then the other. The hand giving the treatment should be very relaxed. Support its elbow with the other hand to hold it in position. If this isn't possible, an alternative is to treat the back from the front at the same height. In this case, be sure to give about 10 minutes of Reiki instead of 3 minutes.
13. Place your hands horizontally on the lower ribs at the height of the kidneys so that two fingers rest beneath the ribs.
14. Let one hand rest horizontally on the sacral plate above the behind, with the other vertically beneath it, below the crotch (body contact is not necessary since Reiki is also effective through the aura). The root chakra can only absorb larger amounts of Reiki when the area beneath the base of the spine (coccyx) is treated.

The Leg Positions

15. Let the hands cover the backs of the knees. When giving yourself a treatment, it is more comfortable to place your hands on the front of the knees. It is very pleasant and increases the effect if you first treat one knee with both hands—one in front and one in back—and then treat the other knee in the same way.

The head positions (1-5)

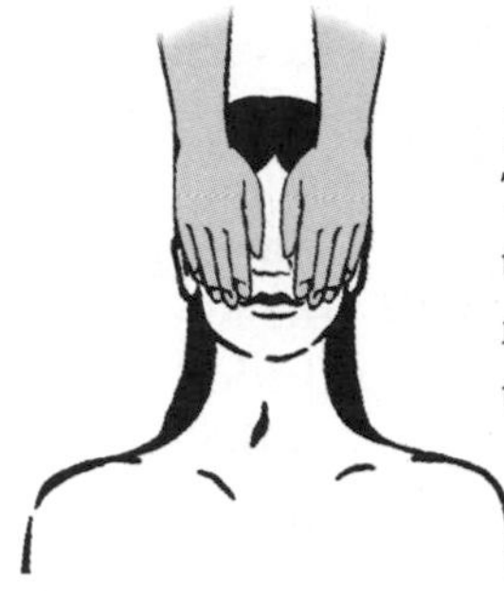

1.
The hands are placed to the right and left of the nose, from the forehead to the eyes

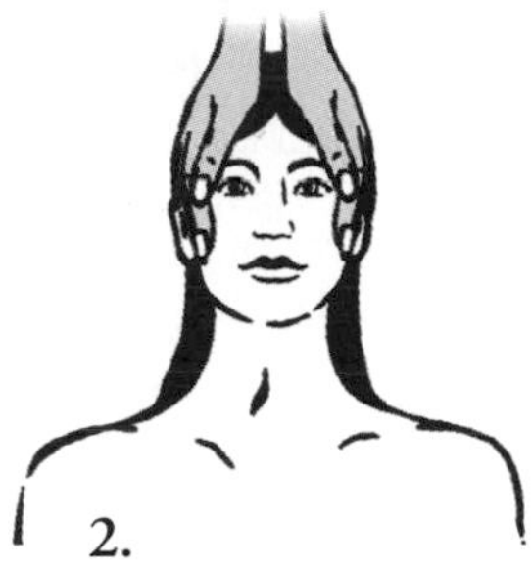

2.
The hands cover the temples

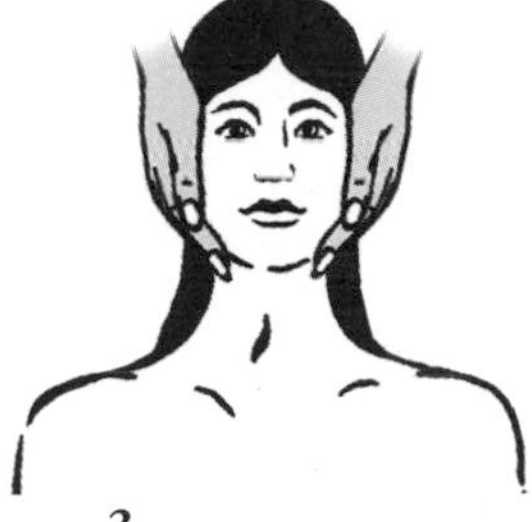

3.
The hands cover the ears

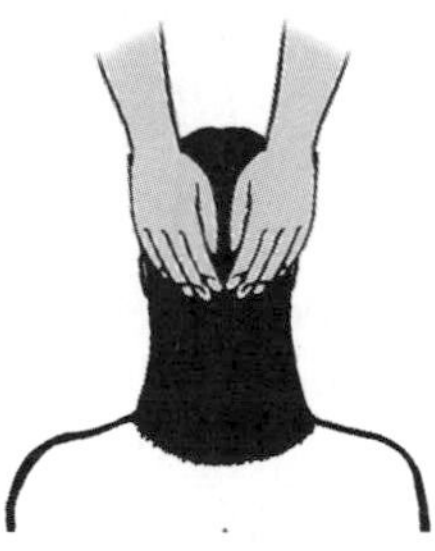

4.
The hands are placed on the back of the head

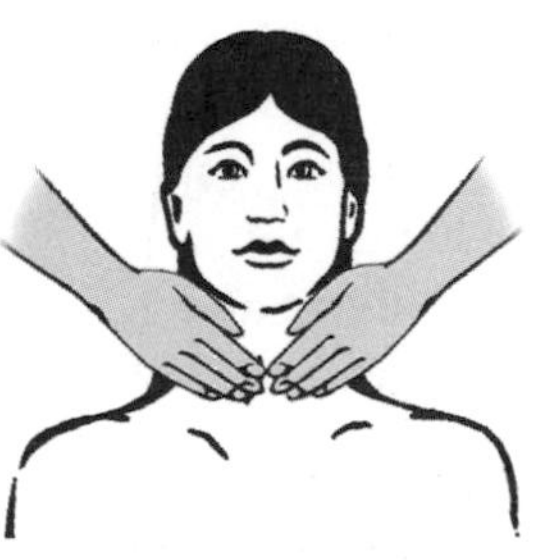

5.
The hands cover the throat

The trunk positions (6-10)

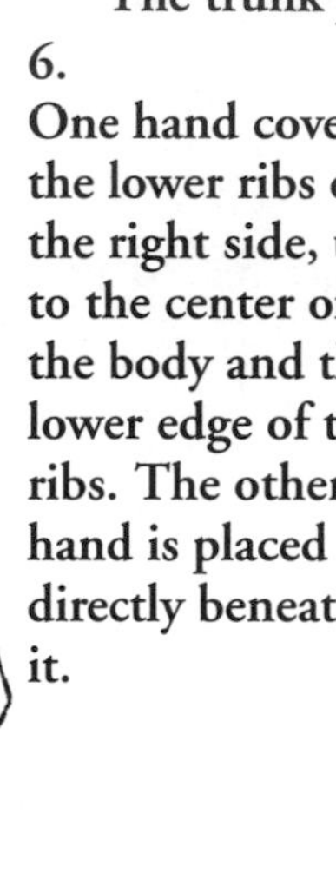

6.
One hand covers the lower ribs on the right side, up to the center of the body and the lower edge of the ribs. The other hand is placed directly beneath it.

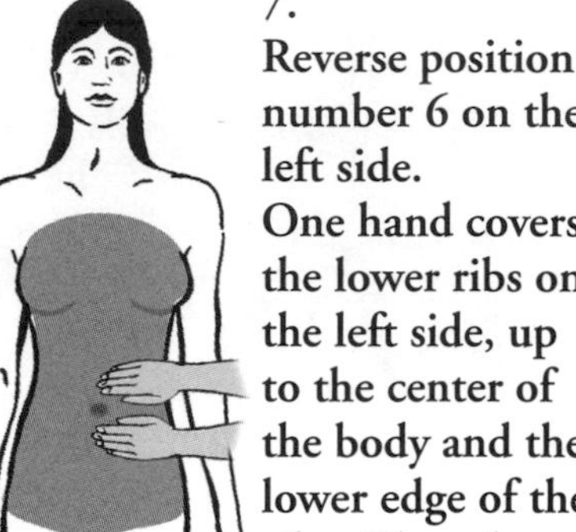

7.
Reverse position number 6 on the left side.
One hand covers the lower ribs on the left side, up to the center of the body and the lower edge of the ribs. The other hand is placed directly beneath it.

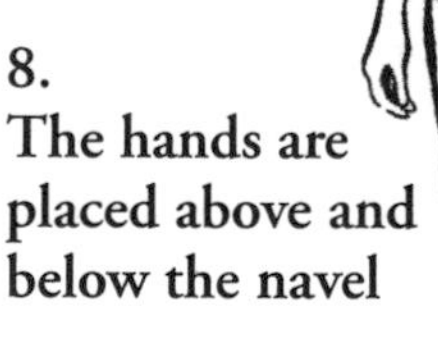

8.
The hands are placed above and below the navel

9.
One hand is placed directly below the throat horizontally on the thymus gland at the center of the body and the other vertically on the heart area

The back positions (11-13)

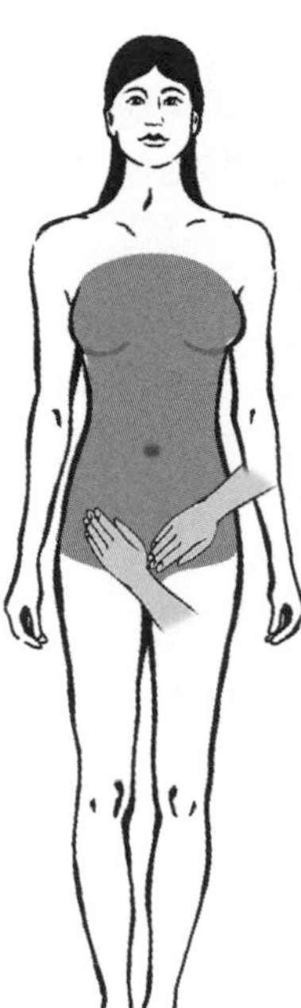

10.
Beginning with the somewhat protruding pelvic bones to the left and right on the upper pelvic area, the hands are placed so that they reach the beginning of the pubic bone.

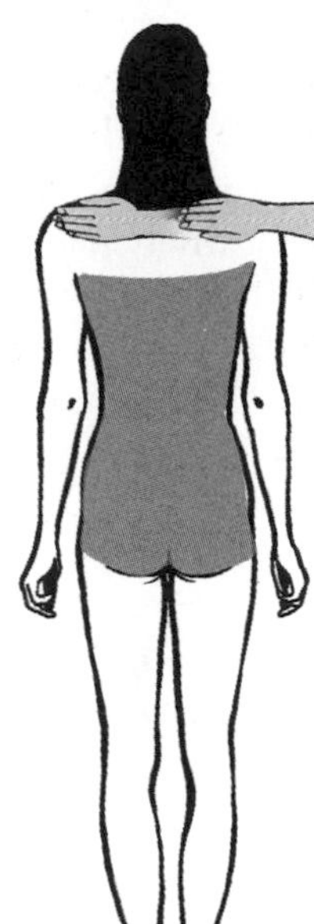

11.
The hands are placed horizontally between the upper side of the shoulder and the shoulder blades to the right and left of the spinal column

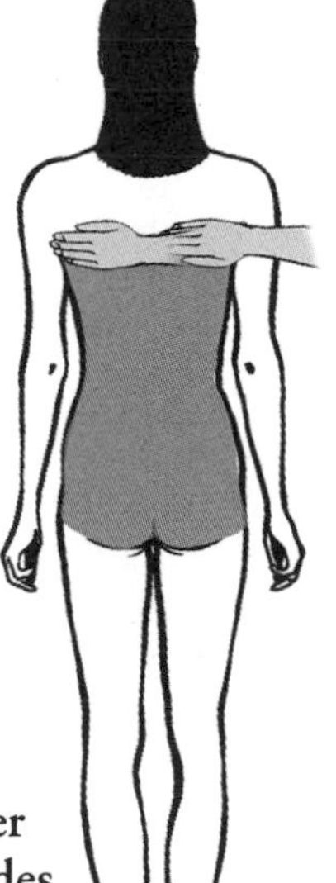

12.
The hands horizontally cover the shoulder blades

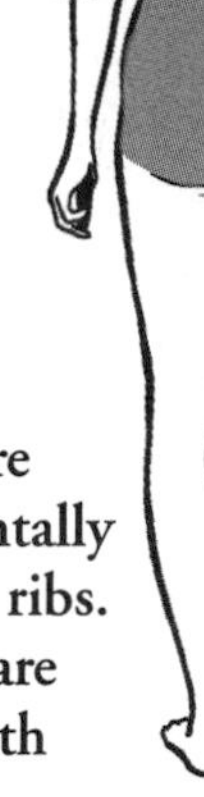

13.
The hands are place horizontally on the lower ribs. Two fingers are placed beneath the ribs

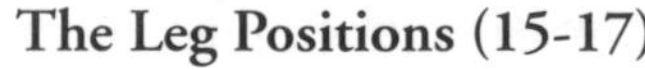

The Leg Positions (15-17)

14.
One hand rests horizontally on the sacral plate above the buttlocks, with the other vertically beneath it

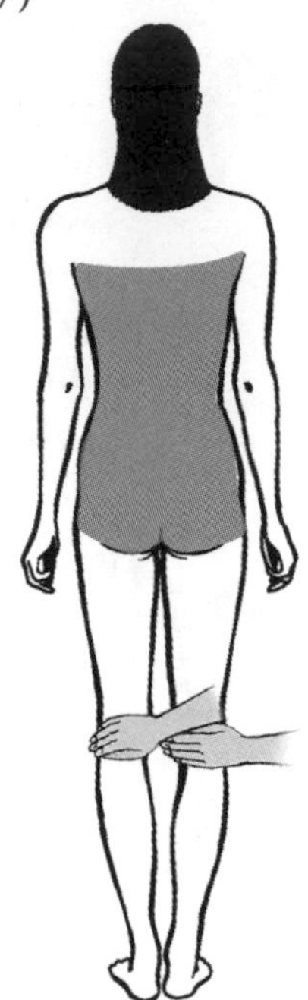

15.
The hands cover the backs of the knees

16.
The hands are wrapped around the ankles

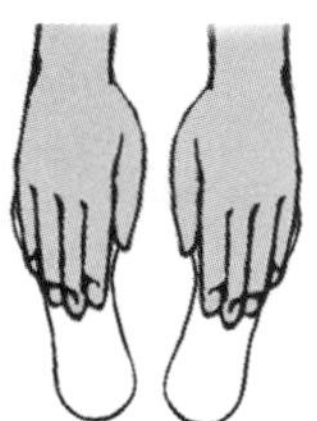

17.
The hands are placed on the soles of the feet, from the toes to the middle area of the feet

16. Wrap your hands around the ankles. It is very pleasant and increases the effect if you first treat one ankle with both hands and then the other ankle.
17. Place your hands on the soles of the feet, extending from the toes to the middle of the foot; be sure to cover the big toes.

The Correct Conclusion of the Treatment

- As at the beginning, smooth out the aura at least three times. However, you should place one hand above the client's sacrum this time. It is possible to make a reflexive contact with the client's hara through the sacrum.
- Ask if the client feels well and has a clear head. If this is not the case, treat the knees, ankles, and soles one more time with Reiki. A light massage of the legs and feet also helps against grounding problems.

In some individual cases, a sense of unwellness and head symptoms may occur within the scope of a Reiki treatment because toxins and waste materials are being released from the inside of the cells in the physical area. These enter the blood, lymph, and interstitial fluid, which means that these substances must now be eliminated by the detoxification organs. Blocks in the energy area are also dissolved. The body's own energy system normally releases these energies into the earth through the legs and feet. However, if sizable blocks still exist along this path, these problematic forces cannot leave the body and create disharmonious symptoms.

- In addition to the tips listed above, it is helpful to end the treatment of the joints with Reiki by drinking several glasses of water charged with Reiki, as well as rubbing the joints, diaphragm area, and chest musculature with sweet almond oil that has been previously charged with about 15 minutes of Reiki. Further possibilities for grounding are: dancing, garden work, sports, sex, washing dishes, eating, bathing the feet in alternating warm and cold water (caution: should not be used on people with heart problems or high blood pressure!), and walking on the ground with bare feet.

If everything is in good order, conclude the session by bowing with your hands folded in front of your heart. Give thanks for being allowed to be a Reiki channel.

Explanations on the Positions for the Whole Body Treatment

The individual positions that are used within the scope of the whole body treatment all have a deeper meaning. The order of these positions is also in no way coincidental. Their meaning is explained in the following section.

The client's aura is smoothed before the whole body treatment in order to:

- Create a personal, energetic contact between the treatment-giver and the client's body consciousness.
- Attune the treatment-giver to the client and the treatment situation.
- Cleanse the aura of energies that are superfluous at this time and impede the natural metabolism. This also strengthens the aura's natural functions (in essence, these are: shielding from disruptive influences, communication of energies, temporary storage of outside energies that currently should not (completely) reach the inner energy system and of energies from the inner system that should not be (completely) released to the outside world.)
- Promote the ability to absorb Reiki and the release of disharmonious energies from the client's inner energy system to the earth through the aura.
- Provide a first impression as to the location of congestion and blocks. These become noticeable through "sticky," "cool," or intense tingling sensations. When the hand glides over a larger block in the aura, a perception of something coarse may arise. Bad cases of trauma may also be felt as strong sharp pain in the hands of the person giving Reiki. In order to harmonize the unpleasant sensations in your hands; shake them a number of times to the earth direction. In stubborn cases, place your hands on the ground for a moment and ask Mother Earth to draw all the energies out of your body

that don't belong to it. Then release the disharmonious forces symbolically in the form of a dark cloud into the earth through your arms and legs with each exhalation. However, these procedures are rarely necessary. Even at the level of the First Degree, anyone who has been properly initiated into Reiki will already have very extensive protection against taking on the client's disharmonious energies during a treatment. After all, everything that comes from the client must ultimately pass through the Reiki field radiating from your hand and finger chakras. In this process, disharmonious energies are transformed so that nothing harmful is usually left to "backwash" into the treatment-giver.

Note: A calm, gentle, and slow movement is helpful for becoming attuned to the client—similar to Tai Chi Chuan.

The technique of smoothing the aura treats the central channels of this energy field, which are located about one to two handbreadths above the center line of the body. Their direction of flow runs evenly from the top of the head to the feet on the front and back-side of the body.

Explanation of the Effects of the Individual Whole Body Treatment Positions

1st Position

The *6th chakra is strengthened in its functions* in order to better direct the energies in the inner and outer energy system that begin to flow later in the treatment in a holistically meaningful way. This is an absolute precondition for intensive healing. This energy system coordinates the harmonious cooperation of all the cells, organs, and function systems in the body, as well as attuning the person's way of living in the outer world with his or her plan in life and the constructive, harmonious interplay of the various personality aspects.

In addition, this creates a balancing effect on the stomach meridian, which runs from the area of the solar plexus over the chest, neck, and face through the eyes and shifts the activity of the brain more to the front section, the zone for freely associating consciousness. Through the better functioning of the stomach meridian, problems can be processed more effectively and creative solutions for difficulties on all levels can be found and translated into reality. The resistance to stress is improved and self-perception indirectly strengthened. According to the perspective of Traditional Chinese Medicine, without a well-functioning stomach meridian no healing reactions can be triggered. If, by way of exception, an individual does not react to Reiki even in a continued, correct treatment, you can make an attempt to give Reiki to the larger area of the stomach and the entire course of the stomach meridian. This often distinctly increases the willingness of the organism to heal.

This is one of the two key positions for the whole body treatment. The second position is no. 17 at the other pole of the body.

Among other things, this position treats: the 6th chakra; the frontal, maxillary, and paranasal sinuses; eyes and teeth; various reflex zones and acupuncture points, including the stomach meridian; as well as the neurolymphatic reflex zones of the stomach meridian on the frontal eminences.

2nd Position

This balances the two brain hemispheres so that the feelings (right) and the intellect (left), the head and the belly, work more closely together. This means that the following developmental processes triggered by Reiki do not remain one-sided and are accepted and supported by both sides. Balancing the brain hemispheres improves the overall self-healing and learning abilities, as well as the holistic approach to life. It becomes easier to relax and the ability to concentrate is also improved.

The secondary chakras located on the temples regulate the flexibility of the vision and the ability to assume and tolerate various standpoints and perceptual perspectives with our consciousness. This supports the development of a more holistic way of evaluating and judging situations.

Among other things, this position treats: the two brain hemispheres, the nerves and muscles of the eyes, as well as the nose/throat area and the temple chakras.

3rd Position

Through the acupuncture points of the ears, the entire body is prepared for the direct application of Reiki in terms of the reflex zones. This exercises very gentle healing stimulation on all of the organs and systems, increasing the body consciousness' ability to absorb Reiki and direct healing stimulation.

In addition, the equilibrium organs and parts of the brain—above all, the general integration zone*, which controls human behavior in stress situations according to fixed patterns—the opportunity of receiving Reiki. As a result, the behavior programs that are resorted to under intense stress and are no longer appropriate can more easily be attuned to the needs of the present by the body's own mechanisms of reorganization. Moreover, the perceptive abilities are improved and relaxation promoted. In most cases, the following principle applies to Reiki treatments: the gentler they are, the more effective!

Among other things, this position treats: the outer ear with various reflex zones for practically every area of the body; inner area of the ears, parts of the brain, and the equilibrium organs.

4th Position

The normalization of many unconscious body functions is promoted through the *medulla oblongata*. This prepares the organism for the material level of the healing process and the release of blocked energies. In the area of the medulla, the 6th chakra is connected with the other main energy centers through the spinal-column channels of ida—sushumna—pingala. In these places, Reiki promotes the 6th chakra's unimpeded exchange of information with the rest of the energy system so that the organizing impulses of this energy system

* The general integration zone is located about two fingers above and behind the ears.

are properly directed on to the body and the organ's feedback can be correctly received. In this position, the area of the brain that regulates the body temperature receives Reiki.

In addition, the head reflex zones for the body areas extending from the head to the pelvis are supplied with Reiki, reaching the upper area of the cervical spine.

An acupuncture point located in the area of the medulla has a very relaxing effect. Many people doze off during this position. Please be sure to let them sleep and simply continue the treatment!

5th Position

The 5th chakra is strengthened in its functions so that the client can more easily let go of blocked energies and release them to the outside world, as well as harmonizing his or her habits, in this position.

The neck is also the link between the head (intellect) and the trunk (emotion), as well as between the structure-giving, organizing (yang) and the energy-giving, action-taking authority (Yin). These two poles must meet in order to create true liveliness, the ability to develop, and holistic healing. If the 5th chakra is not functioning adequately and suffers from blocks, the body and mind cannot work together in the proper manner.

The better this chakra functions, the more relaxation is possible since tensions can be released in an appropriate way. Needs that may become conscious can be better articulated. *The 5th chakra is the first "organ" that is treated to promote the release of subtle energies.*

Also compare the bodily function of the thyroid gland and the parathyroid gland in this respect.

Further important functions of the 5th chakra are related to the entire speech apparatus, artistic and esthetic talent, and mediality, as well as the individual expression of the divine spark that is embedded deep within every human being and begins to radiate more and more through a spiritual way of life, having an effect in the outside world through the material form. Clairvoyants can perceive this in the form of a very clear and warm aura.

Among other things, this position treats: the energetic center for communication and self-expression (5th chakra/energetic element: ether), thyroid gland and parathyroid gland, vocal cords, larynx, and some of the lymphatic nodules, as well as the ganglia that are located in the carotid artery and are responsible for the regulation of the blood pressure.

6th Position

Now treat the liver, another materially oriented organ, in order to use the possibilities of improved organization created by previous specific Reiki applications to Positions 1-5. If we first supply the liver with Reiki but do not strengthen the energy-directing possibilities (Positions 1-5) of the body, the powers of self-healing would not necessarily be completely activated. This is because the large amount of released energy cannot be directed meaningfully in this situation. In relation to the body's biochemistry, as well as the energetic processes of the control directions, the liver is also dependent upon instructions from above—meaning chakra 5 and, above all, chakra 6.

By stimulating the liver/gallbladder function, Reiki can help to release the blocked driving forces, as well as improving the digestion, detoxification and removal of waste materials, general resistance to stress, and overall vitality. For the additional positions, it is absolutely necessary that more energy and an increased ability to shape an appropriate lifestyle are available. A well-functioning liver provides the body with strength and the mind with the powers of assertion and motivation to take action. For example, people who have a hard time getting moving in the morning often suffer from a weakened liver function. Depression and depressive moods frequently have their physical basis in disorders of the liver function.

Among other things, this position treats: the liver and gallbladder (physical: detoxification, digestion, metabolic processes, energy exchange), a portion of the ascending large intestine, a portion of the stomach, the tail of the pancreas, a section of the transverse colon, and the portion of the 3rd chakra that is related to the organization of the digestion in terms of breaking down the food, with the nervous system, the vision, and the various types of headaches (through the connection with the stomach meridian that runs through the eyes) that are related to fears, a sense of power, and helplessness, as well as practical thinking.

7th Position

Immediately after strengthening an organ for the release of energy (liver and gallbladder), the energy organ responsible for directing these forces—the spleen*—is provided with Reiki in order to ensure that the energies of the liver are used in an optimal manner.

On the physical level, the spleen is also responsible for removing phlegm from the organism—meaning the removal of proteins that can no longer be used physiologically. This is why it often plays a large role in the naturopathic therapies against cancer. Moreover, by treating the pancreas,** as well as indirectly preparing the treatment of the energetically related main chakras 3 and 4.

The energies mobilized in Position 6 must soon be directed into the proper channels so that they can have the greatest possible benefit. In addition, for the first time there is a harmonizing effect on the ability to have relationships (through the pancreas and its connection to the 3rd and 4th chakras), which plays a large role in the following positions. Incidentally, the elbows are an important reflex zone for the pancreas, which can be well-provided with Reiki as special positions for all pancreas problems.

Among other things, this position treats: the spleen, pancreas, descending large intestine, a section of the transverse colon, and a portion of the stomach.

Practice tip: If you intend to treat the pancreas in particular, be sure that the recipient of the treatment has an empty stomach. Otherwise, Reiki will partly go to the stomach and its contents instead of into the pancreas unless you treat it for an extended period of time.

---

* The largest lymphatic organ; important function in the immune system, removal of phlegm from of the body, and direction of the liver energy to the other organs, as well as the translating it into practical actions; brooding, doubting, pondering, and lacking charisma in a blocked state; realization of the energetic potential through realistic decisions and actions in the functional state.

** Physical level: on the one hand, important digestive functions through the production of digestive juices; secondly, the control of cellular glucose absorption by producing the hormone insulin. Energy level: unification of analysis/synthesis; connection to the 3rd chakra with its themes of digestion, power, analysis, setting boundaries, self-perception, ego function, and fears. Also includes the 4th chakra with the themes of social environment and integration into groups.

8th Position

Reiki for the abdominal region, including the hara (center of a human being's equilibrium and connection to certain spiritual energy sources) and the 3rd chakra, strengthens the ego function of the body, as well as its abilities to set limits and digest in every sense. It also supports relaxation, the feeling of being centered, inner peace, the ability to deal with emotional stress, and the vital force in general. In this position, energies are mobilized and the flow of energy in the abdominal area is stabilized. These specific effects are important because the subsequent positions increasingly involve closeness, opening up, and relationships; people can develop serious problems when they cannot adequately open up and set boundaries in a constructive, harmonious manner.

Key words: The "no" comes before the "yes"!

Among other things, this position treats: The stomach/solar plexus (3rd chakra/energetic element: fire) and the transverse colon above the navel, as well as the hara, which is our energetic and mechanical center, as well as our interface with infinity, and the small intestine. There are many reflex zones for the various abdominal organs in the area around the navel.

9th Position

Now it is time to strengthen the heart center with its ability of accepting and creating resonance, saying "yes," opening up to groups, and becoming devoted to tasks and other people. The functions of setting boundaries against qualitatively or quantitatively harmful influences, which were promoted by the last position, provide the necessary foundation so that the individual can become involved with others. After setting boundaries, the theme is now opening up and being together with other human beings on the social and mental level as preparation for the physically oriented involvement and devotion that is promoted and harmonized by the following 10th position.

The pelvic region is generally burdened with the greatest taboos. This is why the power of the heart must be supported directly before treating this region with Reiki, making it possible to also more lovingly accept this area of the body and its functions such as elimination, reproduction, playing, and pleasure.

Among other things, this position treats: the thymus gland—which is very important for the functioning of the immune system on the physical level. In energetic terms, it summons the power of the liver into the body. The thymus gland is important for youthfulness, vitality, and physical and mental freshness. It can be activated by tapping it lightly on a regular basis, followed by an application of Reiki. There is a connection between the heart and the thymus gland. Here is a rule of thumb: If the heart is healthy, the function of the thymus gland is also strengthened. Reiki at this point is also good for the heart and bronchial tubes (related to the lungs), as well as the 4th chakra with its themes of love, the ability to accept, family, synthesis, and social responsibility. The heart chakra is associated with the energetic element of "air. " The heart is a big pump that rhythmically moves the blood through the body. The ganglia above it create a type of built-in rhythm generator for the heart. The heart therefore creates the frequency in which it works. Although this can be changed externally through the brain, only the heart can make itself beat. If we move in harmony with our own heart rhythm, we are in harmony with ourselves; our movements are esthetic and flowing, such as those of a master of Tai Chi Chuan. If we move against our own heart rhythm, our movements will appear to be choppy and unaesthetic. The more we act in disharmony with our heart rhythm, the more our heart rhythm becomes strained. In the long run, this may even cause damage to the organ.

The lung is *the ultimate* exchange organ with the surrounding world. An individual's attitude toward the natural process of give and take is formed here, as well as the way in which a child has received love from the parents, especially the mother. If a child is bound to a relationship with an apparently loving parent and forced to behave and adapt in a specific way, lung disorders such as asthma are more likely to develop in the course of time.

The body's supply of oxygen and fresh vital energy from the air, as well as the disposal of carbon dioxide and vital energy that the body no longer can use, is regulated through the lungs.

10th Position

When Position 9 has strengthened the function of accepting, including "accepting ourselves" and the harmonious exchange with the surrounding world on all levels that is based upon this acceptance, then treat the pelvic area with the 2nd chakra. In the Western culture, this area of the body with its eliminatory, reproductive, and primary pleasure organs tends to be treated as shameful or is aggressively rejected instead of being loved from the heart. This leads to extensive and sometimes very complex problems particularly in the area that has a central significance for the development of vital strength and joy in life, as well as creativity and a deep feeling of connection with other beings on a physical level. Strong and very stubborn blocks frequently exist here.

Among other things, the 10th position also includes the greatest creative possibilities of a human being: the ability to reproduce with all of its associated energetic and material function systems. Furthermore, the motor of a human being is located in the 2nd chakra, which puts us in the position of accomplishing the greatest achievements—and having fun while we do so. This motor is the joy of living, playing, and creating, and the joy of encountering other individuals. In contrast to the "starter," the will (which causes us to be self-disciplined through the conscious decision of taking action, has the task of tearing us out of our natural sluggishness in order to ensure our survival and advancement through meaningful actions), pleasure and joy can make it possible for our body, mind, and soul to achieve wonderful accomplishments in a relaxed, long-term, and very effective manner.

The area of the pelvis is therefore associated with great energies that make it possible to take action, survive, and experience a deep connection with other people. However, that's not all; the eliminatory functions are at home here in the deepest part of the trunk, which is closest to the Earth. Only through elimination can we let go to a large extent of what impedes us, what torments us and can destroy us from the inside out if we don't free ourselves of it. Feelings of guilt that we have not yet healed, for example, are located in the large intestine. The large intestine has a certain connection to the lungs and is very important for the function of the lymphatic system and the body's defenses.

Body therapists have known for decades that proper work with the reflex zones, musculature, and connective tissue through massages or influencing the life energy with methods like Reiki causes the digestive system to become quite active.* The organs involved in the digestive process not only digest material substances but also information, feelings, and the related energies. The process of digestion integrates everything that is useful to the organism and eliminates everything that is harmful or impeding to it. The more poorly the digestion functions, the less the afflicted person will be strengthened by everything that has been absorbed, causing the outer effects to be a greater strain on the body. Good digestion and elimination are vital for an individual to be strong, healthy, and self-confident in the most positive sense.

If the stuck energies in the 2nd chakra in particular and pelvic area in general are stimulated to flow more quickly and become very strong through Reiki without the appropriate preparations,** there may possibly be a renewed stronger splitting of these forces through the body's defense system, which may not be prepared for the integration of these forces. Through careful treatment of all of these energy centers that are important for the integration of these strong vital forces, it is much easier to guide the released energies appropriately and effectively.

After this central functional area has been strengthened, the treatment can be continued on the back side of the body. This is where the more strongly suppressed experiences and energies of a human being (shadow aspects) are stored.

11th Position

Assuming responsibility and "nourishing" other people is only meaningful when this is done in a way that is playful, pleasurable and in harmony with our own developed ability to be in relationships, and

* The effects described here are called *psychoperistaltic.*

** For example, through very long treatment of this position, together with specific chakra work in combination with healing stones or through a very strongly developed sensibility and intense energy congestion.

appropriate to our own physical nature. With Position 9 on the heart and lungs and Position 10 on the 2nd chakra, these preconditions are improved, at least for a time. Nourishment and responsibility are the themes of the secondary chakras that are connected to the energy channels of the spinal column between the shoulder blade and the shoulder. They extend toward the front through the chest and open into the aura and the outside world. When an infant is breast-fed by the mother and she is fearful of or disgusted by her own physical nature, the little human being often receives a very problematic double message: "I am nourishing you and feel disgusted or fearful as I do it."

Nourishing others either psychically or physically so that their individual needs are appropriately meet is only possible when we can focus on our own individual being and lovingly acknowledge it. We can never give others what we spiritually deny to ourselves!

Responsibility has various meanings: On the one hand, it makes long term relationships possible, especially under strained circumstances. Consequently, it is the foundation for the social network on the basis of mutuality and a sense of security. On the other hand, responsibility is the key to leadership, healing, and teaching qualities. However, there are two main problems in dealing with responsibility:

- We basically do not want to assume much responsibility because we feel inadequate. At some point, usually during childhood, we have learned that we must be perfect when we do our tasks. If we don't succeed in this, there's no point in even trying. This belief is naturally the greatest detriment to learning! Absolutely everyone who learns makes mistakes. If we try to learn from our mistakes, get back on our feet again, and keep going—we will succeed.
- We want to assume a great deal of responsibility and achieve as much as possible because we are convinced that this is the way we will receive love and attention from others. But this is almost always an erroneous conclusion. No matter how much we accomplish—at some point, even an unusual performance becomes something normal. Then the praise becomes less and less frequent. This leads in increasingly higher standards on our own capacity. Sooner or later, the inevitable result will be excessive strain and—in the extreme case—collapse. But there is an additional major error involved in this ap-

proach. The value that a *function* has and the value of a *person* have little in common with each other. If we want to be loved as the people we are, we must seek others who do not judge us according to the criteria of achievement, who want to play and share enjoyment with us in a great variety of ways. This allows us to experience human closeness, understanding, warmth, loving affection, and the feeling of security in the relationship with each other.

Being successful in every way and becoming familiar with our own possibilities (and boundaries), slumbering talents, and concealed potential through challenges that we create for ourselves is certainly an important aspect of life if we want to be fully awake. But performance and success should never become a criterion for human values—otherwise, we will soon find ourselves in an ice-cold robot society.

In terms of the order, this position is also very important because it improves the connection of the head and trunk in terms of energy, nervous system, and muscles through the back of the body.

Moreover, after the area of the 3rd chakra with its supporting organs (Positions 8-10) have been extensively provided with Reiki, it is possible to harmonize important storage depots of this function bearer in the shoulder area (secondary chakras of nourishment/responsibility) that must intercept things that are "indigestible" and other strains from the outside. If the secondary chakras of nourishment/responsibility overfilled with the fears, frustration, and feelings of powerlessness that the 3rd chakra has passed on to them in order to better maintain its own ability to function, tensions in the shoulder and neck can easily develop. This is naturally also possible because of the reasons explained above in detail or through a combination of causes. An important rule of thumb: If there are more intensive blocks or strong symptoms in the area of the nourishment/responsibility chakras, the 3rd chakra should also receive a large amount of Reiki since there is quite a strong probability that it has contributed to this problem.

Near the prominent cervical vertebra (that sticks out somewhat) at the level of the shoulder, there is a type of energy pumping station consisting of a secondary chakra in the spinal column and the acupuncture points that work together with it, the *Upper Pakua*. This point provides the head and throat area, shoulders, arms, and upper back with the strength that the chakras make available to it. In the case of intensive fear, spasms or cramps can occur here that prevent clear thinking and remembering (such as blackouts during exams; "losing your head" in critical situations).

Here is a little practice tip on this topic: Many people with these types of symptoms have been helped by taping an amethyst (about the size of a cherry) that has been charged with Reiki for about 20 minutes to the Upper Pakua. Over the course of several hours, this will usually visibly improve a person's stability.

12th Position

This is where the flow of all the feelings is stimulated by the effect of Reiki on the acupoints of the bladder meridian on the skin and kidney meridian about two to three fingers beneath the skin, and the lungs. Furthermore, important points of the small intestine meridian—which regulates the absorption, transformation, and distribution of energies and nutrient components—also receive Reiki.

Now the lungs take in Reiki again, which further stimulates their functions of accepting and releasing. The heart and the heart chakra are also treated again with this position. In this context, it is perhaps interesting to once again give some more precise thought to the functions of these two organs: during their entire lifetimes, both of these organs must work without interruption: both are set into operation through muscles, and both are associated with the energy absorption and release processes, as well as with the creation of relationships. The lungs take in energy and air from the surrounding world and release energy and air that has passed through the metabolism in the body to the outside world.

This makes the continual contact between the inside and the outside possible. If the release or absorption (meaning the cycle of eternally changing energies in the system of life) is interrupted for a longer period of time, the human being will die.

The individual's relationships with the outside world are essential to life—in the spiritual sense as well! With its right chamber, the heart is closely connected to the lungs. The blood is pumped from the right chamber through the lungs to the left heart chamber. Among other functions, the blood releases its carbon dioxide and absorbs oxygen from the respiratory air. It's no coincidence that the right side (the yang side of the heart) is essentially available to the lungs, which is the organ oriented to the outside world, while the left heart chamber is responsible for the inside of the body as the yin pole.

Just like the lungs regulate central areas of the body's relationship to the outside world and, with their own rhythm, can provide an adaptation of the heart's rhythm to the outer vibrations, the heart represents an orientation for the entire body's own vibrations through its rhythm. By way of the blood, the heart provides for the constructive relationships of the organs and cells with each other. Both organs, the lungs and the heart, do not actually process what they transport. Instead of evaluating things, they provide a steady flow of the forces and information, attuned to the inner and outer rhythms of life. If a person has mental or emotional problems of a serious nature with this principle, organic problems may result in time.

Another important effect of this position is stimulating the body armor (which we know of from the field of bioenergetics), causing the chronic tension of the muscles to "melt away." However, it is only meaningful or even possible to gently dissolve congested emotional energies or cause them to flow away after extensive preparation through the previous Positions 1-10 and, above all, 11. When the body cannot process these, it will simply attempt to freeze them or make others responsible for their resolution according to the motto of: "It's your fault that I feel so terrible!" Growth and healing in the holistic sense are very much impeded as a result of this attitude. If people feel very rigid—like a tree trunk when you hug them—or the other extreme of rather limp and cold, this position is very advisable. If possible, this position should be provided with the universal life energy for a much longer period of time in each session.

The 12th position is also used as a preliminary position before the direct treatment of the large "flow center," the kidneys, since the 13th position promotes the functionality of the responsible distributors and channels of the energy element of water. It empties the storage areas that are responsible for the non-integrated "conflictual" energies.

13th Position

The kidneys are the bearers of the individual relationships to other beings, the hereditary forces, blood purifiers and energy suppliers for many areas of the lower back, the arms, and the legs. Together with the 2nd chakra, they manage the element of water in the organism. Now they can be stimulated in their complex diversity of functions. The ability to have relationships with others has already been strengthened in particular by Positions 5, 10, and 12. Prepared in this manner, it becomes easier for the kidneys to fulfill their tasks to a greater degree. They are not just dependent on their own energies, but are supported by the energy centers and channels associated with the kidneys. This is especially important for the kidneys as relationship organs. Above all, the heart and lungs are important "working colleagues" of the kidneys in both the physical and energetic sense. This safeguards the kidneys from becoming exhausted too quickly, which can happen particularly in cases of long-lasting major strain, negative stress, or a lack of interpersonal support.

Before strengthening and harmonizing the earth forces (root chakra, leg and foot positions), it is useful to first completely provide the essential functional bearers of the water energy with Reiki. Otherwise, the body doesn't know what to do with such an improvement in its grounding. This grounding absolutely requires the body to "be in flow." In addition, the strengthening of the water element in the body is an important precondition for energetic detoxification and removal of waste materials through the legs and feet, then down into the earth.

Because of its relationship to the adrenal glands, which are located above the kidneys and are associated with the 1st chakra, this position is very important for regeneration and constructive stress management. Anyone who tends to have cold hands or feet should additionally receive at least 15 to 20 minutes of Reiki in this position as a special position within the scope of the whole body treatment. This rule of thumb applies here: *The kidneys* tend to be responsible for *cold hands* and the adrenal glands for *cold feet.* Both are very closely related to fears. Cold hands show fears related to the physical and emotional contact with others, while cold feet indicate that the respective person generally is afraid of having to master life alone and *independently* as an adult.

In conclusion, the relationship between sexuality and the kidneys should be mentioned: The kidneys suffer when there has been an imbalance between sexual wishes—especially those that have been triggered by outer influences—and their satisfaction.

In the psychic sense, kidney stones and renal sand develop through unloved feelings, such as physical tenderness and sexuality in relationships, as well as chronic fears—which are usually associated with the above states. Suppressed anger and constant stress in emotionally significant relationships increase the tendency toward inflammatory disorders of the kidneys and its functional field.

In acute cases of *paralysis* and problems created by fright and shocks of all types, the kidneys are an important special position that also shows good results when treated with Reiki. People who react as if *paralyzed* because of a longing for the past standing in the way of the present, and/or have difficulties in opening up to closer relationships, can receive important help toward a healing orientation in the here and now through intensive Reiki at this position.

In order to function well, the kidneys require an adequate supply of water. The minimum is 30 ml of non-carbonated water per kilogram (2.2 pounds) of body weight every day. Alcoholic drinks, soft drinks, fruit juices, milk, and milk drinks count just as little toward this amount as coffee or black tea.

Many people, especially older individuals, suffer from a chronically reduced feeling of thirst. This is the result of the bladder meridian, which runs in two branches to the left and right of the spinal column through the entire back, being filled to the brim by suppressed feelings. Individuals in this situation should be sure to drink the amounts of water stated above, even if they do not experience a feeling of thirst. A normal feeling of thirst often arises in time if this is done. Furthermore, the back can be treated with Reiki, handbreadth by handbreadth. Stroking it with a rounded crystal quartz that is at least the size of a walnut, previously cleaned with cold water and then charged with Reiki for about 10 minutes, can also be helpful.

For more serious problems with the kidneys, always include the 2nd chakra, also giving it some extra portions of Reiki.

Pregnant women may have fewer problems during pregnancy and an easier delivery if they are given Reiki on the kidneys on a regular basis since the kidneys provide wide areas of the pelvis with energy. Sciatica problems during and after pregnancy can also be effectively prevented in this manner. As the "organs of closeness," the kidneys endure a great deal during the months of pregnancy because the mother must deal with the closeness of the child.

14th Position

Now the body is adequately prepared for the flow of more extensive energies through the activation of the energetic element of water in the two previous positions. Consequently, the 1st chakra—as the body's own strongest source of strength—can now be given Reiki. Since a "power plant" with an enormous potential of archaic energy—which also includes the kundalini energy—is now switched to full speed here, give Reiki to the *Lower Pakua* (a type of secondary chakra that provides the lower back, the pelvis, and the legs with the energy of the chakras, as well as linking the 1st and 2nd chakras with the inner energy system through the energy channels in the spinal column).

This approach ensures that vital forces do not congest in the pelvic area; instead, their vitalizing influence is available to the entire body. The center of the human being that organizes all of the forces associated with the energetic element of water is located here.

When the water forces flow more intensely, they need the earth forces to balance their activities, just like a river receives its natural course through the structure of its bed made of soil and rock. Without this "grounding," water cannot produce any kind of liveliness. A strengthened connection to the earth force outside of the body can now be created. The concluding positions are responsible for this function.

Among other things, this position treats: the sacrum with its energy pumping station (the Lower Pakua) that supplies the entire abdominal and pelvic area with strength; the 1st chakra (survival, fight and flight, structure, blood, vitality, bones) is stimulated. This position is also well suited for strengthening and treating disorders and/or disharmonies of the above-mentioned areas, as well as general grounding.

When a person is very exhausted, wants to recuperate from longer periods of illness, or desires to learn how to better deal with the above themes of the 1st chakra, this position should be treated frequently and for longer periods of time.

It is also suited for the acute treatment of hemorrhoids. However, hemorrhoids—both internal and external—should primarily be treated through the abdominal and pelvic positions. It may also be helpful to drink water that has been charged with Reiki to improve digestion and confront the guilt feelings that burden the large intestine as well as holistic treatment to improve the metabolism of connective tissues.

15th Position

Energy easily becomes congested in the large joints. Since the entire inner energy system is grounded through the feet and legs, meaning that the body draws fresh strength and draws off forces that are no longer useful for it into the earth through them, it is very important to keep these joints free of congestion. An old Chinese proverb says: "healthy, strong legs—healthy, strong person!"

The large joints are easily blocked in terms of their energy. On the physical level, they are also frequently a type of "final disposal site" for the body when it cannot eliminate or transform certain intolerable substances into some other form. This creates deposits in the joints that impede their functioning. On the path from the trunk to the earth and back, the flow of energy can easily be blocked. This is especially true since the themes of the knee chakras, "teaching and learning," can also be quite a problem for many people. Foot treatments with Reiki or massages have a much better effect when the large joints (ankles, knees, and sometimes also the hips) are energetically harmonized beforehand.

In general, all problems related to teaching and learning, feelings of inferiority, excessive pride, arrogance, inadequate optimism, and associated themes respond well to treatment with Reiki. When dealing with these themes, it is absolutely necessary to consider the connection of the knee chakras with the 3rd chakra and also give it an extensive treatment. The effect of Reiki treatments on the secondary chakras is often greatly intensified when the associated main chakras also receive Reiki.

People who play ball sports such as football, soccer, volleyball, or handball can tolerate large amounts of universal life energy in this position because the knee joints are very strained through the many vehement turning motions.

16th Position

As the next largest joint on the way to the feet, the ankles should be given Reiki so that the stream of energy can also flow freely here and grounding isn't blocked. With the Positions 14*, 15, and 16, the preconditions are created for the concluding position to have an optimal effect.

The ankles and their surroundings are reflex zones for the abdominal and pelvic region. Moreover, they contain secondary chakras that are responsible for an individual's ability to flexibly create the conditions for personal survival, as well as being able to provide for his or her livelihood, security, and well-being under unusual or quickly changing circumstances. These secondary chakras also support trust in our self-preservation skills. Keep this attribute in mind and also treat the main chakras 1 and 2 with an extra portion of Reiki.

17th Position

All of the energy channels are now activated through the reflex zones located in the soles of the feet—especially in the front area up to about the center of the arch, which is responsible for the upper area of the body. This activation is only possible when no larger areas of congestion exist in the leg joints. If this position is used individually for the harmonization of dizziness, headaches, migraines, or general energy congestion in the head and throat area and results in either no effect or very little effect, the reason is usually energetically blocked leg joints. In this case, give several minutes of Reiki to the knee and ankle joints—Positions 15 and 16. For stubborn cases, also treat the

---

** In addition to the effects discussed above, in Position 14 Reiki also ensures that the sacrum is relaxed and congested energies can flow away.

hip joints through the greater trochanter. This will eliminate the energy blocks. After this has been done, the treatment through the soles of the feet will also function much better.

This position is naturally suitable for grounding, the balancing of the energy flow within the body, harmonizing and strengthening the aura, as well as support in the treatment of the 1st chakra.

Number 17 is a general position that can be successfully applied for every treatment purpose, in as far as it is extended to the entire sole of the foot and the upper area of each foot and ankle. One way of greatly intensifying the effect is to gently massage the feet with a light touch and calm, stroking, and circular motions—possibly with a bit of naturally pure massage oil.

The whole body treatment with Reiki is concluded by way of this position in order to allow the blocks that Reiki has dissolved in other areas of the body to flow down to the earth; it can also be used to create a counter-pole for the strong yang charge in the yin area, balancing the energetic flow as a result.

People often speculate why the leg and foot positions probably did not play such a significant role for Mikao Usui and Hayashi. In my opinion, this can be attributed to the following circumstances: During this era in Japan, there was much less of a tendency toward grounding problems because of a lifestyle that was generally quite earthy in comparison to that of our modern society. Be that as it may, grounding techniques have quite a few positive benefits and allow so many problems to be solved that they should definitely be part of every Reiki treatment repertoire.

This position treats: reflex zones for the head and throat, the kidney meridian (acupuncture kidney 1), and the solar plexus point in the front area of the feet. Many reflex zones for the entire body are located on the soles of the feet.

Please note: If an individual is very weak or has grounding problems, a very effective treatment may be to just give Reiki through the feet.

If excessive healing reactions occur either during the course of the treatment or at some point afterward, Position 17 usually offers quick help and guides the disharmonious energies into the right channels.

Smoothing out the Aura at the Conclusion of the Treatment

Smoothing out the aura at the end of a Reiki session has the following effects, among others:

- Dissolving the energies that have flowed out of the inner system into the aura and are still stuck there. When the aura is stimulated to flow, energies that are intolerable for the body can be released to the earth.
- A conclusion of the treatment process on the emotional level and a harmonious parting of the partners
- A general benefit to the functions of the aura, which meaningfully supports the inner energy system in its tasks.

Some tips for the practice:

a. If it is very difficult to get the aura flowing, you can put a little bowl of salt about two handbreadths beneath the client's feet. Salt has an intensely cleansing effect. However, the salt should only be used for a few minutes before, during, and after the aura has been smoothed. Salt binds any type of subtle energy. When it has drawn out the easily dissolved, inappropriate energies in a living system, it will begin to bind the vital forces. Especially in the open state during an intensive Reiki session, a person can then easily yield some of his or her own energy. But if you follow the above instructions, you won't have to worry about this. In case of doubt, immediately remove the salt if your client has the feeling of being weakened or disharmoniously influenced in some other way. The salt must be flushed down the toilet after the session. It should absolutely not be used as food for people or animals or poured onto plants!

b. In many cases, the effectiveness of the treatment can be greatly increased if you smooth out the aura frequently during the session and then continue with the positions. By doing this, you will help your client more easily release the energies that are problematic for him or her. Smoothing the aura will also make it easier for the client to open up to Reiki because the aura can more freely accept the beneficial influences from the outside world as a result. The aura can also be smoothed in the individual areas. Always be sure that you smooth it over the arms and hands or the legs and feet.

After the Session

After an extensive Reiki session, a nap of 15 to 30 minutes is very advisable—it intensifies and deepens the effect. During the nap, it is good to keep warm for the following reason:

The body knows two phases of fundamental energy distribution. When it is important to work, to act, or to deal with the outer world in some way, the vital energy is increasingly gathered in the musculature and skin. In these areas, the circulation is also intensified. When it is important to recuperate, digest, regenerate, relax, and heal, the vital energy is directed to the inner organs and the digestive tract. Consequently, the body cools down easily during the second phase and it is important to keep it warm so that the precious time of regeneration and healing is not ended too quickly of necessity or a cold and/or tensions develop.

Conversations about the experiences during the treatment, except when it appears to be absolutely necessary, should be held after the session and the nap so that the ensuing process is not disturbed.

With the exception of most acute cases, *the success of a Reiki treatment* cannot be often seen directly during or shortly after a session but in the gradual, constant change toward health and liveliness in the client's everyday life. This process is similar to the one observed when a constitutionally oriented homeopathic treatment is given or when Bach Flowers or Californian Flower Essences are taken as a harmonizing influence upon problematic habits and character structures.

Lacking, weak, or very intensive energy experiences during a session indicates *nothing* about the effectiveness of the treatment. In other words: If the client doesn't notice any sign of Reiki during the treatment, this absolutely does not mean that Reiki has been ineffective. In this case, it works outside of the respective person's perceptive possibilities.

About the Special Positions

The following applies for all of the special Reiki positions:

- Treat on a regular basis and at least 15 to 30 minutes per position, at best within the scope of a whole body treatment or in addition to regular treatments. In difficult cases, you can use these special positions several times a day over a longer period of time!

- A special position may be any position of the whole body treatment or applied to any other area of the body that either shows symptoms or is connected with the symptomatically conspicuous area through an interaction (reflex zone).

Reiki is not the same as acupuncture, shiatsu, or reflex zone massage! Reiki is not concerned with recognizing and treating the "right" place. Instead, it is primarily important to give Reiki to the *entire* body so that its systems can function better and it can heal itself. As a supplement to this, and in acute cases, the special positions[28] are obviously quite useful.

There is a simple rule of thumb for when the whole body treatment is appropriate and when the special positions should be used instead: If symptoms are acute and occur only on a limited area or part of the body, the individually applied special positions are generally adequate. For example: one single burn blister or an insect bite without any further complications or a headache, as long as it does not occur on a more frequent basis. The whole body treatment is generally the remedy of choice if the symptoms are distributed widely throughout the body, such as the following: sunburn on the back, legs, and belly, psoriasis, cancer, or AIDS. This also applies if they have a definite psychic origin such as the effects of a shock, fear, or stress. An additional category is chronic symptoms such as asthma for the past ten years, neglected infections, and headaches that occur on a regular basis[29]. However, supplementing the treatment with the special positions can usually greatly improve the effect.

Individuals without health problems can use the whole body treatment as an intensive method of holistic personality development. In this type of application, it is interesting to keep a journal on the experiences during the treatment of the individual positions and compare your notes with the explanations of the positions. In this way, for example, it is easy to become familiar with ourselves on the deeper levels and receive impulses for specific types of character development.

The Treatment of Burns, Injuries, Infectious Skin Disorders, and Similar Problems

In some of the illnesses afflicting the skin, any type of touching is felt to be very unpleasant or even painful. In such cases, treat the client at a distance of one to two handbreadths above the surface of the body. Moving the hands in a gentle, calm manner can intensify the treatment.

Power Intensification in the 1st Degree

Unfortunately, too few people know that some very effective techniques of power intensification can be applied even in the 1st Degree of the Usui System of Natural Healing. Incidentally, these can also enormously intensify the effectiveness of almost any type of treatment in the 2nd or 3rd Degree.

The "homeopathic" touch:
Almost without touching them, *very gently* massage the zones that you would like to treat for somewhere between 20 seconds and 2 minutes. Then lay your hands on them as usual. According to the Arndt Schulze Rule (from the field of biocybernetics), fine impulses stimulate life activities while strong ones inhibit them. The fine impulses of the massage technique explained above direct the attention of the body consciousness to the appropriate area and intensify the body's perceptive abilities. At the same time, the receptivity is increased. Prepared in this manner, Reiki is absorbed at a much higher degree.

Aura massage:
Calmly hold your hands about two to three fingers above the area to be treated for about 20 seconds and attune yourself to it. Then let the hands begin to move gently. Be sure that the palms are always facing your client's body. After about 20 seconds, again hold your hands calmly for another 20 seconds and attune yourself. Repeat this technique several times, then treat the position as usual. By relaxing the aura, the possibilities of energy flowing to the body are improved because Reiki clears the aura. In addition, through the fine

impulses of the aura massage, the attention of the body consciousness is directed to appropriate places. This, in turn, increases the receptivity. *Wherever the attention is focused, the energy will flow more freely in that direction.*

Blowing on an area:
Hold your hands so that they face each other and are about two handbreadths apart. For a few seconds, hold them at a distance of about two to three handbreadths in front of your mouth. Then gently blow between your hands several times toward the body area to be treated. In this way, Reiki will reach the inner energy system of the body more easily through the Ki contained in the breath, intensifying its receptivity. After blowing on it, treat the position as usual.

Singing vowels:
During the treatment, sing the vowels A, E, I, O, U, and M. This stimulates the chakras and the aura to gently increase their vibrational level. The higher the vibration of a being, the greater the willingness of its organism to absorb Reiki.

Rubbing hands:
Shortly before the beginning of the Reiki treatment, lightly clap your palms together and rub them intensely for a moment. This stimulates the hand chakras, through which Reiki is transmitted, to more intensive activity.

Baby oil:
Rub your palms with a few drops of baby oil. During the treatment, be careful of sensitive clothing and treat within the aura, if this is possible! I can't explain why this technique functions so well, but it is widespread among faith healers and has great results.

Tip: These six techniques can naturally also be combined with each other.

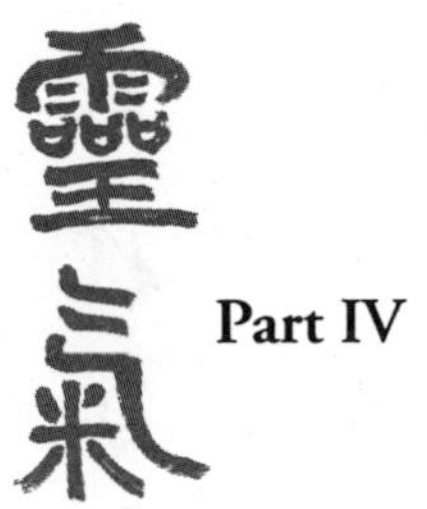

Part IV

REIKI TODAY AND TOMORROW

われもまたそらにみがかむ曇なき
人の心をかがみにはして

: 125 ***The Mirror***
I should polish my self
More and more
To use the others' clear
And shining heart
As a mirror

CHAPTER 21

Walking the Reiki Path

Working with the Life Principles in Theory and Practice

—by Walter Lübeck—

On the one hand, the Usui System of Reiki is a very effective method of holistic healing through the transmission of universal life energy (Reiki) from one person to another. On the other hand, it is a completely valid route of spiritual personality development, a mystic path to the light.

As a healing method for the body and mind, Reiki requires as its basis the participation in the appropriate initiations and training in the use of spiritual life energy. This training includes the following, among other things: the whole body treatment, aura work, intuitive Reiki, harmonization of the chakras, special positions for the specific treatment of certain health disorders, as well as rules for a healthy diet and a constructive lifestyle.

However, if you would like Reiki to bring harmony to your soul and guide you on the path to the light, something else will be necessary: knowledge about the mystic aspect of the Usui System of Natural Healing. Up to a few years ago, very little was known about this in the West. But through intensive research, a significant amount of which was based on the work of Frank Arjava Petter, it was possible to also shed light on this foundation of Mikao Usui's lifework. In addition to the life principles, the central themes of the mystic path of Reiki include meditation, the esoteric meaning of the Reiki symbols, and the *waka* that Mikao Usui used to teach his students; these are spiritual didactic poems written by the Meiji Emperor, who Mikao Usui greatly valued. This chapter is dedicated in particular to the meaning of the life principles and how to use them for personal work.

My involvement with Reiki as a spiritual path began in 1987, shortly after I had participated in a First-Degree Reiki seminar on a beautiful weekend in spring. Some days later, it occurred to me that I could not literally translate the life principles into action, even though their meaning and significance were completely clear to me on an intuitive level. So I began to search for a way to use the life principles in a practical manner and become informed about their philosophical background. This was the beginning of a long process of learning, growing, meditating, and trying things out, probing, and thinking. I am certain that I have not reached the end of this process. This isn't even something that I want to do since I feel that the path is the goal—and attaining the goal is just one phase before a new segment of the path begins. But perhaps the things that I have experienced and tried out with my friends and students will help you progress a bit further with Reiki on your personal path to the light.

The Life Principles and Mystic Aspect of the Usui System of Natural Healing

To me, writing about Mikao Usui's life principles also means telling something about the mystic aspect of the Reiki path—Reiki Do. Less familiar than the active aspect—with its colorfully dazzling variety of symbols, mantras, hand positions, chakra work, mental healing, aura harmonizing, distance healing, and much more—this quiet realm only opens up to those who are truly willing to look into the clear mirror of the divine self. This is the divine power of meditation and contemplation, devotion, insight, and understanding. As a result, in the sense of the ancient Asian yin-yang philosophy, it complements the more active (yang) side of treatment methods and techniques, making it possible to apply the universal life energy with the yin perspective.

During the first years of my involvement with Reiki and Mikao Usui's heritage, I was very confused by the greatly differing versions of the life principles. Many Reiki Masters were quite emphatic about representing their opinions, which strongly deviated from each other, and the available books didn't offer a genuine clarification. Although each source claimed to be authentic, traditional, and in the spirit of Mikao Usui, no one could actually prove this since there was practically no free access to the source material for this topic at that time. "Supplemented" or "modernized" formulations of the Reiki life principles appeared time and again. We can be certain that they were based on good will and the desire to help; however, modernized versions teach us nothing about the path that Mikao Usui discovered. This is only possible through the original principles.

While I developed contacts with other Reiki friends, read esoteric books, and telephoned or corresponded with various Masters, I increasingly had the impression that many people were moved by the life principles, but no one really knew what to do with them. Apparently, many people—just like myself—were attempting to make the best of these five short sentences, but did not have the original material available to them. A Reiki Master who I met at the beginning of the 1990s had a very simple "solution" for this problem: "Always orient yourself on the life principles and don't think so much!" Although this may sound good, I don't know of anyone, including myself, who can simply turn these life principles into reality. This is where things became difficult.

The situation changed abruptly when I finally had access to Mikao Usui's original life principles and his written statements about his teachings as the founder of the Reiki method through Frank Arjava Petter. With great enthusiasm, Arjava and Chetna had already been researching the history of Reiki for a longer period of time. They had found Mikao Usui's grave and much written material by and about him. The two of them discovered the life principles in the inscription chiseled into a large monolith on Mikao Usui's grave at a Buddhist cemetery in Tokyo.

The original life principles have now been published in the form of the original Japanese text, as well as in translation, in the books by Arjava. Here are the five Reiki life principles:

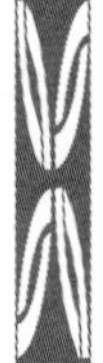

1. *Just for today don't get angry*
2. *Just for today don't worry*
3. *Just for today be grateful*
4. *Just for today work hard*
5. *Just for today be kind to others*[30]

Mikao Usui did not develop these simple rules on his own. He got them from the Meiji Emperor, who ruled Japan at the turn of the 19th Century. The Meiji Emperor opened up Japan for the West and strove to give his people a spiritual orientation. Mikao Usui used some of these Waka, a special form of poetry, in his Reiki seminars to explain important spiritual wisdom to his students, letting it come alive through the poetry.

The life principles assume a central position in his heritage, as far as we know today. What is so important about these five sentences? What help can they give us on the spiritual path taken and taught by Mikao Usui, which millions of people throughout the world today follow either directly or indirectly?

In order to truly understand the essence of the life principles, we must first trace them from their apparent, exoteric message back to their esoteric, spiritual content. The next step is to understand the practical application of these five sentences. I would also like to include some of the approaches that have proved to be very useful in my work here.

The Hidden Message of Mikao Usui's Life Principles

If we understand the life principles in a literal manner, they cannot be translated into practical terms. Instead of helping and healing, some of them would even create blockages in the long run. Anyone who actually attempts to never be annoyed or worried, always work hard, be thankful and loving to others, will end up as the GHS (Great Hypocritical Suppresser) or become frustrated and cynical or depressive at some point because of his or her presumed failure.

Didn't Mikao Usui know anything about these easily comprehended effects? Was he a superman or did he want to convey something deeper with these strict instructions than is obvious at first glance? As we know today, the founder of the Reiki method saw a great deal of the world. He was apparently aware of the esoteric use of the language. If a student was to be stimulated to personal development through principles and texts, the content would have to be formulated in such a way that the meaning is complex and the individual messages are only discovered through precise study, as well as the basic questioning of everyday thought patterns. The life principles are short and to the point—but as full of meaning as an average library. Naturally, this cannot be completely explained in detail here.

But we can take a closer look at some of the central insights. Are you ready to take a little journey to the mystic Land of Reiki?

The Meaning of the "Here and Now"

To explore the mystery that the Meiji Emperor and Mikao Usui have left for us, we can examine the individual life principles to see how they harmonize with each other. Perhaps they have a mutual theme.

One important quality is shown in the recurrent repetition of the word "today." This unmistakably points to the importance of the present moment. All significant spiritual teachings agree that human beings can only be truly happy, love, discover who they are, feel the pulsation of life, develop their talents, and take action for the good of all in the here and now. Only in the present moment do we have the opportunity to influence our situation in life and change it for the better. If the greater portion of our attention is focused on the past or the future, we will not be as successful or learn as much when it comes to surviving both the everyday and the unusual challenges of life as those who are in the present moment with their consciousness. We will also naturally have less fun.

The key to the secret of spiritual awakening can be found in the here and now. This is the key to the firmly closed door that separates the realm of love and light from the material world. Letting the "self" completely blossom in the present automatically results in the personal ego entering into the Great Divine Light. Mikao Usui was aware of this truth. After his 21-day period of meditation and fasting on Mount Kurama, a famous holy place for centuries in Japan, he had a profound experience of enlightenment. This experience empowered him to create the Usui System of Natural Healing from the knowledge, experience, and abilities that he had collected during his lifetime. Then he passed them on to other people.

Accordingly, a fundamental message of the mystic path of Reiki is "Be in the here and now with your consciousness. This is the only way for you to come to the Great Divine Light. This is the only way for you to change your life for the better and give it a more spiritual meaning."

As we now explore other aspects of the wisdom concealed in the life principles, please always remember the fundamental orientation described above: The awakening in the here and now is the basis for a genuine spiritual consciousness, as the flexible channel for the divine power that flows through individuals who are awakened. Through them, it flows into this world and is capable of supporting healing and peace, happiness and development.

1. Anger Can Be a Tremendously Positive Source of Power

The first principle deals with the power of aggression, the vital life energy that also has its home in the root chakra of the human being.

Mikao Usui says: "Don't get angry!" When properly understood, this message can open up a vast source of power. Anger is the way in which aggressive energy expresses itself when it is short-circuited, meaning that it is separated from constructive action. When we feel anger within ourselves, we should get to the bottom of this feeling as quickly as possible and clarify the purpose for which the Higher Self has sent this powerful energy to the body and mind at this moment. Then we should think about how this power can be meaningfully translated into actions and get to work. In my experience, anger or annoyance stops as soon as the hidden intention of the energy activated at that moment is turned into a meaningful action: As a result, the underlying need experiences satisfaction.

The individual steps of this somewhat complicated procedure are naturally only necessary until a new habit and expanded consciousness have been created and old blocks that stop us from taking action have been healed. A helpful aid in this process is the Reiki Gassho meditation, which was rediscovered in Mikao Usui's writings by Frank Arjava Petter and has a special connection with the practical application of the life principles. In order to practice this meditation, sit on a chair or meditation cushion, place the palms of your hands in front of your heart, and focus your attention on the tips of your middle fingers.

Every moment spent in a meditative state is naturally time well spent. However, it has been my experience that the deeper-reaching effects and spiritual experiences can only be expected after practicing daily for at least 30 minutes on a regular basis.

Moreover, Reiki mental healing with selected affirmations on the specific harmonization of blocks in our actions, as well as Reiki meditation with the healing amethyst gemstone, are useful. These are described in detail in my *Complete Reiki Handbook*.

In this deep spiritual healing process, it is enormously important to discover the actual cause of the anger. For example, when we become angry because of another person, we should not rest until we have understood what has triggered our *own* fears and what unpleasant qualities the other person is actually displaying. If we become annoyed about something on the news, a scene in a film, or an article in the newspaper, it is good to find out—in objective terms—why something so distant from us and sometimes even fictional should concern us personally. We can reflect upon what we truly fear—since fear is always connected with anger—and which (perhaps suppressed and unloved) parts of our own personality have risen more intensely into our conscious mind through what we have experienced. If this important healing process does not take its course, talks with a personal spiritual advisor, meditation on a regular basis, and intensive oracle work are very helpful.

This is the first life principle. When you work with it, you can heal and develop your root chakra. The power of this energy center is enormous and the challenge great. Summarized into one question, it says: "Would you like to continue to be angry and complain about others—or do you want to energetically get to work on turning the truth, beauty, and goodness in this world into reality and thereby let the divine work through you to your best knowledge and conscience?"

This life principle can set the power free upon which the subsequent life principles depend in order to function for us.

2. Worries Can Be Harmonized, Just Like Anger

In a certain respect, worries are similar to anger. Meditation, contemplation, intuition, conversations, and oracles can help us find the actual, real, and personal reasons. This allows us to translate the basic energy caught in the worries and fears into constructive, meaningful actions, which will ultimately free us. Worries show that an aspect (usually unconscious) of a human being feels it is losing control over significant things necessary to survival or maintenance of important resources. In other words: The subconscious mind believes that things could soon become quite dangerous, painful, or somehow uncomfortable, and doesn't know how to remedy this situation at the moment. Then we feel worried. But we can solve this problem when we know exactly *what* we fear. In most cases, in the light of consciousness the cause of the fear turns out to be unreal or can be dissolved with a little bit of effort. So we can look in the dark corner and notice that no monster is lurking there, or run away in time, effectively defend ourselves, negotiate, or positively influence the situation in some other way. Reiki can help us in a particularly effective way when we direct our attention to the worries, giving ourselves three to five minutes of Reiki at each of the six lower main chakras. While doing this, the hands should not touch the body but remain at a distance of one or two handbreadths from the body. As a result, Reiki can more easily reach the respective energy center.

This life principle deals with the power of fear. If we take a closer look at fear, we can see that it is just a guardian, but many people make it the ruler of their lives. When fear is put in its proper perspective, the power of the root chakra is no longer suppressed. Its energy becomes available to us on our personal path. Fears tell us: "Stay where you are! Don't move! Make yourself smaller than you actually are!" Reiki tells us: "Recognize your strengths! Get up and walk your path in your own way! Set a good example for others, especially those who are weaker, and help them find their personal path and take it seriously!"

Working with this rule heals important areas of the 2nd and 3rd chakras.

3. Gratitude Creates Basic Trust and Connects Us with the Rest of Creation

Gratitude means recognition of the special grace, the divine blessing received in everything that is given to us, no matter how small or large it is. Nothing that life gives us is a foregone conclusion. The streams of energy from the divine can flow to us—or sometimes they don't. Our personal achievement is minimal when related to the enormous effort that life engages in to nourish each of us with all that we need. Practicing gratitude means connecting ourselves with the network of life and, supported by it, attaining the power of basic trust. When we are thankful, we acknowledge the greatness of the creative force. We also acknowledge the divine spark of its power, which lives within every human being and lets our heart-beat, allowing the body and mind to live. Gratitude creates basic trust. Based on the repeated practice of gratitude, only the growing awareness of the caring presence of the divine can diminish the feeling of being alone and having to fend for ourselves in a life that we feel to be hostile. The source of life invites us to a feast, which is meant in both the literal and the figurative sense. Gratitude makes us successful. How often do people overlook the helping, giving hand of the creative force because they insist upon a *very specific* type of happiness and success. They base this demand on the opinion that they always know what is best for them or even because they don't understand what else could be there for them. Gratitude sharpens the sense for understanding divine influences. In the chakra theory, this effect can be associated with the sixth chakra at the center of the forehead.

This life principle helps us avoid ending up in isolation. Only those who are conscious of the connectivity of all life can truly perceive the divine. No matter who we are, where we come from, and how things are going for us at the moment—we can call upon the grace of the creative force, use whatever is necessary, and start improving our situation. The source of life offers enough nourishment for everyone. We don't have to fight against others for things to go well for us. We can fight for ourselves and take a stand for those who are weaker if we have some strength left over. We should pray for help, be attentive, and give thanks for what we receive. If we accept this from our hearts, we will understand that the right things will always come to us at the right time.

4. Working Hard on Ourselves Helps Us Overcome Stubborn Resistance and Become Familiar with Our Own Powers

Many people experience the challenge of "just for today work hard" as a provocation since we more or less live in a democratic leisure-time society, which tries to escape the "dictatorship of work" by means of all types of distractions. This work may be uncomfortable, but, realistically speaking, a spiritual calling can actually only be translated into reality by means of quite difficult, long-term work. But no one said that this work shouldn't be fun and personally meaningful.

It's quite amusing to imagine that, after eight hours of work on the spiritual path, Jesus or Buddha said they had the evening off and didn't want to deal with the stress until the next day. Or that during his weeks of meditation on Mount Kurama, Mikao Usui got up from his meditation cushion punctually at 5 p. m. every day, shook out his legs, and prepared for his leisure-time activities. *Work in the spiritual sense is primarily and foremost work on ourselves.* Only when we do it in the proper way—and incessantly—can we increasingly open up to our divine self. This hard work is not drudgery imposed by someone else. It is only necessary because the well-trained habitual patterns of fear and greed, a sense of separation and envy, jealousy, and hate, self-doubt and unconsciousness, self-denial and irresponsibility will otherwise seize rulership over our path in life and destroy the healing success that has been arduously achieved through love, attention, expansion of consciousness, and devoted, meaningful actions. During his meditation on Mount Kurama, Mikao Usui was only able to follow his calling and totally turn it into reality because he did not let himself be restricted by the 8-hour workday or the 35-hour working week.

Today, some people tend to judge their profession as if it was basically unspiritual. They make idols out of their distractions. Yet, this does not create happiness, fulfillment, or self-love in the spiritual sense. This approach is not meant to turn workaholics into the true saints. It is also important to make genuine rest and relaxation possible through this hard work on ourselves. Not being able to *truly* relax is a widespread health disorder in our age: In our thoughts and feelings, we are torn back and forth between the fear of missing out on something or being punished for "laziness" on the one hand; on the other hand, we are afraid that by relaxing we will get too close to ourselves and no longer be able to adequately suppress the unpleasant things that we might discover. A certain amount of effort is required to heal ourselves from these types of bad habits. In this sense, hard work means making the serious effort to walk the path to God, for example, in the here and now and not just twice weekly at a meditation class for two hours. Only this type of steadfastness can lastingly dissolve and harmonize the blocks that prevent us from reuniting with God.

This healing path naturally also includes relaxation. Yin and yang can be found everywhere—even here. However, the work related to our occupation or profession should not be shortchanged in this respect. Not everyone works as a seminar coach, personal advisor, or guru. If this were so, the disadvantage would be no more breakfast rolls and missing bus drivers, no one working at the cash register, and no one who could repair a broken appliance. In my opinion, spirituality is only meaningful when it can be translated into everyday reality and thereby enriches everyone's life. In this respect, our occupation or profession includes our calling as the spiritual dimension of the work with which we earn our livelihood. If we do not seriously involve ourselves in our work, working hard on ourselves within the scope of our work and filling out our place in the world as well as possible, then we cannot find the way to ourselves during our working day and we cannot take our own path. This means that much time is uselessly wasted, lost, and "gone with the wind. " Like relationships and everything else in life, work should be taken seriously, enjoyed, and carried out in a playful manner. Then we can let our talents come to life and develop our strengths—and others will benefit from this as well. When we consider our occupation or profession as our calling, then we will do good work and treat our business partners and customers the way they deserve to be treated: as the people who make it possible for us to take our path to the light.[31]

This life principle reminds us to truly get involved in life, not waste our time, and use our opportunities. There is absolutely nothing wrong with having hobbies, spending time with friends, and having fun to balance out work and other situations that demand a higher level of achievement and responsibility. Yet, it is important not to let ourselves go too much. Our time on Earth is precious since we can only learn and translate certain things into reality here on this planet. The number of admission tickets for this world is limited, and so many angels are waiting in line to receive the opportunity for self-realization in the material world. When we are back "upstairs," there will be plenty of time to rest!

5. The Challenge of Practicing Spiritual Love

Treating each other lovingly is perhaps the hardest challenge of all. Why? True spiritual love wants the best for everyone involved—not the well-meant but ultimately superficial adaptation of behavior. Treating each other lovingly can mean a smile or hug at the right moment, a good word or deed carried out with heart and understanding. But love can also be the determination, clarity, and strength of holding people back from running headlong into disaster until they can come to their senses and calmly make a genuine decision for their future path.

Spiritual teachers are often called upon to prove their love for their students by showing them their blocks and shadows, their self-abnegation and lack of love—and what can be used to heal these obstacles so that the path to the light opens up. They do not always appear to be "nice" to their students in this process—sometimes even quite unpleasant. However, only those who truly love will take a risk for someone else's benefit. And this risk also includes possibilities such as not being liked at times.

This life principle calls upon us to recognize and honor the divine in others. When we perceive the creative force in everything and learn to respect its workings, we can take one step further and recognize ourselves in the many mirrors and feel the flame of life within ourselves. We all belong together since we are all ultimately in the same boat. Time and again, we should reflect upon what this means and understand it on a more profound level. This perspective may appear to be wrong on the surface, but there are also truths behind the scenes where the threads run together. After our departure, we will comfortably sit together with friends and enemies, sipping a double angel tonic, and be wonderfully amused about our past lives on Earth.

Summary

The life principles of the Usui System of Natural Healing are not intended to be understood as a rigid catalog of rules. They are an appeal for us to thoroughly scrutinize our own behavior and give up senseless habits. The life principles are meant to provoke and stimulate us into thinking more about our life. And they are koans, spiritual riddles, like the Zen masters have used for centuries in order to help students put the rational mind, which always wants to control everything down to the last detail but actually knows very little about life, in its place. Ultimately, they are an important aid for the practical approach to Reiki. Here are a few tips:

- Do the Reiki Gassho meditation for 20 to 30 minutes and, either in your mind or quietly out loud, repeat the individual life principle that you have selected for this exercise. After each repetition, try to sense whether something has been evoked inside of you.
- Use the Reiki life principles in Reiki mental healing. This is an old Reiki technique, which is still used today in Japan for particularly difficult health problems.
- Time and again, think about the personal meaning of the individual life principles and take notes on your experience with them, perhaps in the form of a journal.
- The Reiki life principles have many levels of meaning. Some may appear to either contradict each other or your experience in life. But if you truly get to the bottom of them, you will learn to experience the unity beneath the surface of separation. Make the effort, and you will find less separation and more unity within yourself.

The Inner Attitude during a Reiki Treatment

If the above-described disciplines are consistently included in the Reiki practice, some important consequences will result for the Reiki treatment-giver and naturally also for the client.

The Treatment-Giver . . .

Here and Now

- Should strive to completely open up to the treatment situation. No matter what may happen afterward, we can only devote ourselves fully to Reiki and do the right thing for the client with expertise, intuition, and feeling in the here and now.

Just for today don't get angry and don't worry

- Assumes total responsibility for personal anger and worries that may perhaps arise during the course of a Reiki session as a reaction to the client's behavior or that come to consciousness through the Reiki energy field during a session, directing the energies into constructive paths.

Just for today work hard

- Should do Reiki with total devotion while applying it and not see the interaction with the universal life energy as a "nice little leisure-time activity." Continual advanced training in the field, efforts toward personal development, contemplation, and sensing the personal problems of every client, as well as the attitude that Reiki can succeed even—and especially—in bringing healing to this case when the treatment-giver and client work together in the proper manner.

Just for today be kind to others

- Should make an effort to lovingly encounter the clients and give them a sense of being secure and taken seriously. If necessary, the treatment-giver should also be committed enough to address a matter that is unpleasant but important for the client or represent a standpoint that the client may not like but should consider in order to progress.

The Client . . .

Here and Now

- Should make an effort to completely open up to the treatment situation in the here and now. If this is not possible, the client should work together with the treatment-giver—and Reiki to solve the problem.

Just for today don't get angry and don't worry

- Should assume the full responsibility for his or her feelings. If fear or anger arise during the Reiki session, it is good to talk about it and use Reiki to learn to constructively deal with these feelings. It can be helpful to use the technique explained above for giving Reiki to each of the main chakras for three to five minutes. Keep the attention focused on the problematic feelings while doing this.

Just for today work hard

- Can contribute greatly to the success of the treatment when the client gives serious consideration to Reiki, the experiences of the session, and the advice of the treatment-giver, as well as taking the session seriously and not canceling it "on a whim." In the same vein, patience and endurance is necessary for chronic problems or greater disharmonies in life. Reiki can do a great deal but not banish problems that have accumulated through years or even decades of false conduct in one or two sessions.

Just for today be kind to others

- Can be very helpful to the treatment-giver by making an effort to open up in a constructive and loving manner. This principle contributes to a productive atmosphere during the Reiki treatment. When disharmonious feelings desire to be resolved and expressed during Reiki within the scope of healing reactions after the session, it is important to let out what must come out and also think that the people around you are not responsible for your feelings.

I hope that this explanation of the life principles and the related areas of the mystic path of Reiki have imparted some useful ideas to you for your own personal path. You will find more on this topic in the chapters on the Reiki symbol, the symbols and mantras of the Second and Third Degrees.

For Both . . . Be Grateful

Remember that it is not self-evident to have Reiki available, for two people to meet and reciprocally offer each other the opportunity of learning and growing. Our gratitude increases almost automatically when we consciously experience the wonderful effects of Reiki.

CHAPTER 22

Harmony between All Reiki Groups

—by William Lee Rand—

There have been many wonderful things that have happened for Reiki over the last 10 years. Factual information from Japan has been uncovered that validates the free and open practice of Reiki. The location of Dr. Usui's grave and memorial stone has become known and many have had the opportunity to visit them. The Reiki manuals of both Dr. Usui and Dr. Hayashi have been made public, providing us with the original exercises they taught and giving us Dr. Usui's wonderful Reiki philosophy that validates what many have intuitively thought to be true. The popularity of Reiki has grown. The general public is much more aware and accepting of Reiki. Hospitals and clinics are now providing Reiki treatments for their patients, and important legal issues are being resolved. In the next few years, the practice of Reiki is likely to become an established part of our everyday life. Now is indeed the most wonderful time that has ever existed for Reiki on the planet!

An important step in the continuing evolution is for the Reiki community to work more closely together. It is a necessity if Reiki is to remain free. Forces outside of Reiki would like to control it, including other alternative healing groups and government agencies. A strong desire exists to control how Reiki is practiced or even prevent it from being practiced. In Florida, the massage associations have worked to make it a requirement for anyone wanting to practice Reiki to have a massage license. They have convinced the massage board that Reiki is massage! Reiki groups oppose the restriction, and it is likely that it will be overturned. But such problems will continue unless all Reiki people work more closely together. If we do not join together to keep Reiki free, it could be taken away from us.

In addition, a strong Reiki community where all Reiki schools are represented and working with mutual support for each other is a much better position for a positive effect on the local community and the world. A great need for Reiki exists in the world now, and the better we join together, the greater benefit we will be able to offer.

Negative competition between some Reiki groups in the past surfaced, and although it seems to be subsiding, I feel there is still a need to look at the issue. Some have said that their form of Reiki is the only valid form or that their group is the best Reiki group. They have used fear and misinformation to dissuade their students from associating with other Reiki people. Such attempts damage the Reiki community, tend to give Reiki a bad name, and adversely affect the healing available to those involved within the group. It also detracts from the strength and well being of the Reiki community and diminishes the help that can be provided to the community at large.

I focus on the issue because I know it really needs to be dealt with. However, I am also aware of many areas where the problem has been solved or did not exist, and I want to acknowledge those Reiki people for being aware enough and secure enough to have created a vital, loving, cooperative Reiki community.

A well-organized Reiki community made up of many different Reiki groups and schools working in harmony can do so much more than working in isolation. The feelings that can come from being part of such a group are absolutely wonderful.

The tendency not to have loving, accepting feelings toward all Reiki people comes from fear and is not based on any valid purpose. It is also contrary to the spirit of Reiki. Remember, Reiki promotes love, acceptance, trust, and abundance. If one is truly focusing on Reiki, then one can only appreciate other Reiki people regardless of the school or group they are from.

Those who try to use fear and control to increase their Reiki practice get the opposite results from what they want. Such negative qualities actually repel the students they are trying to attract. Yet, their own fear prevents them from being aware of it. The more one attunes to the qualities of Reiki, the more people are likely to be attracted to the individual for treatments or classes. By allowing loving feelings of appreciation to be expressed toward all Reiki people and groups, their Reiki energy will be stronger and they will be healthier and be better representatives of Reiki.

We know that none of us is perfect and that we are on the planet to heal. So be aware that by honestly looking into yourself and working on what needs to heal, you are fulfilling your purpose. By simply improving your own energy state, you are helping others do the same. If you notice any competitive feelings developing in yourself, accept that they are there. At the same time, it is important not to act on them, but to focus Reiki energy on them and allow them to heal.

It is also important to get to know the other Reiki people in your area and work closely with them. Having great friends is one of the gifts of life. Having great Reiki friends is even better. It is worth your effort. Fear keeps people apart; releasing fear between Reiki people can be accomplished if they get to know each other. Exchanging Reiki treatments is a good place to start. You can also talk on the phone or meet in person. If you have a Reiki practice, the improvement in your energy created by being open, accepting of all Reiki people, and actively working together will increase your Reiki business! In order to do this, you need to go against your fears and with the help of Reiki, take action. To begin the process, one must refuse to speak negatively about other Reiki people and refuse to take part in any kind of negative Reiki gossip. It is a very important first step.

A Meaningful Healing Exercise

If such negativity is an issue for you, or even if you think it is just a small problem in your area, here is an exercise that will definitely lead to a powerful healing. Not everyone is able to do the exercise, but with the help of Reiki, it should not be too difficult for most. So I encourage you to go ahead and try. Think about the other Reiki people in your area. Perhaps you know about some of them from Reiki advertising or from an acquaintance. Think about them and if any fear, anger, jealousy, or other negative thoughts come up, make note of them. Then, deliberately think positive thoughts about them. It might be difficult to do, but go ahead and try. As you do this, make note of any resistance you may have. Look at the resistance. As you do so, try to locate an area of your body or aura where this resistance seems to reside. Try to understand what is causing the resistance. Are there specific feelings and if so, what are they? Does any imagery come up, any memories of other people or situations from the past? Then after you have located the area, place your Reiki hands there and send it Reiki. As you heal this internal part of yourself, you will find it easier to have positive thoughts about those you formerly disliked. Remember, even if a person is really negative, your positive thoughts will heal them, not your fear or anger. So it is very healthy to practice such exercises. They will allow you to have clearer insights into others and to accept and value them more deeply.

Many people may say, "Oh, no, not me, I don't have any negative feelings toward other Reiki people." They may be say so because they know they are not supposed to have such feelings and pretend they do not. They may have developed a strong denial mechanism that works almost automatically, so without thinking about it very much, they automatically refuse to be aware of their true feelings without knowing they are doing it, and focus on what they think they are supposed to be feeling as the model Reiki people they want everyone to think they are. So it takes a lot of courage to do the exercise well. One must be willing to admit he or she may not be as completely healed as desired and be willing to do the healing work needed. Your life will take on more depth, and others will have greater respect for you. You will also have a greater appreciation for others and be able to live your life more fully.

Whenever you don't like or have negative feelings toward someone in your outer world, you have the feelings because of something inside yourself you do not like. It is a direct indication that something inside needs to heal. You may find it difficult to accept, but it is true! It takes courage to realize it, so if you are having any trouble, I encourage you to stay with the process. The more difficult the process, the greater the benefit.

In our past, rather than dealing with negative feelings in a positive way, so as to heal them, we began to project them onto others. Often we didn't have any other way to deal with them. We usually projected unconsciously, so we weren't even aware of it. But it is true that the negative feelings we have toward others are the feelings we have toward those parts of ourselves that we do not want to deal with or even know about. We have also hidden seemingly negative aspects about ourselves, thinking no one will know about them and we do not have to deal with them. But they are still present, influencing how we think and act toward others and even attracting people with the same attributes into our lives!

By accepting the possibility that some unhealed state may exist inside and then directing Reiki toward it, you will be healing yourself and improving your ability to relate with others. By doing so with other members of the Reiki community, you will then find it much easier to talk with them and get to know them. By doing this, you will be transforming an important part of your life from an uncomfortable, distressed, fear state into an enjoyable, relaxed, positive state—and everyone will benefit!

Once you are have begun to work on any fears or negative feelings you have toward members of your Reiki community, you will then find it much easier to interact with them, get to know them and begin to work closely with them. Also, once having set this process up inside yourself, if interacting with people in your Reiki community brings up new levels of fear or negativity, a pathway and process will already be set up through which you can access this part of yourself and work with it in a healthy way.

A Heroic Act

Laurelle Gaia was in a Reiki community in Kentucky where the Reiki people did not talk to each other. As she tuned into the situation and talked to a few of the teachers there, she could tell it was because of the fear that there was not enough to go around. The teachers felt that if other Reiki teachers or practitioners set up in their area, they might be taking students from them. They often spoke negatively about each other, hoping that it would convince people not to take classes from the other teachers.

In a health-food store, Laurelle had placed flyers advertising her Reiki classes, only to find them missing the next day. In their place were the flyers for another local Reiki teacher. (We will call her Margaret.) Laurelle had a fairly good idea what had happened, but was willing to suspend judgment. She took one of the new flyers with her and at home meditated on what to do. She sent much Reiki to the situation and soon heard a question very clearly in her mind:

"Are you a teacher or not?" She then realized Margaret did not know about the universal law of abundance.

Laurelle then received help from her guides to write a letter to Margaret. In the letter she explained what had happened to her brochures at the health-food store, without blaming Margaret for it. She also told her about the importance for Reiki people to work together, as it would be a more powerful way to help the public learn about Reiki. She mentioned the universal law of abundance. Then before mailing the letter, she gave it Reiki and said a prayer to heal the situation.

Laurelle then met another Reiki master and the two of them began getting together to share Reiki and to send Reiki to create harmony in the Reiki community.

Three months passed after sending the letter. Then Margaret called Laurelle. Margaret said she had gotten Laurelle's letter, but did not know what to do. She apologized for not contacting her sooner and said she did not understand something in the letter. She wanted to know what the universal law of abundance is.

There was Laurelle's opportunity, created by the guiding hand of Reiki! Laurelle explained that everyone has a place in the universe and that each person has the divine right to receive an abundance of everything good for a person to have. All that one needs to do is to learn how to work with the energy to manifest what is rightfully theirs to receive. After hearing this, Margaret invited Laurelle to a Reiki circle. Laurelle's other Reiki friend went with her.

At the meeting they discussed the need for harmony between the Reiki practitioners in the community. They agreed to work together. They contacted all the Reiki masters in town, including those from different lineages and schools. They set up a meeting at a massage school rather than at anyone's home or Reiki office, so they would have a neutral location. They called the meeting "Harmony in the Reiki Community Healing Circle." Everyone was encouraged to be a leader in some area, such as leading a meditation, presenting a topic, or organizing Reiki exchanges. This meeting evolved into an organization called "United in Healing."

Together they developed a mission statement and held it in their minds as they sent Reiki to it. The group began to grow! They started a newsletter that everyone could advertise classes or sessions in. They began to work together to promote Reiki. They got a booth at a health exposition and took turns throughout the event talking to people and handing out their newsletter and brochures. They did Reiki in hospitals and presented Reiki to various churches. They held an open house with a Reiki talk and demonstration. They conducted Reiki marathons for critically ill people and developed a free Reiki clinic.

As they became actively supportive of each other, everyone's Reiki practices began to grow! Those who were truly able to fill their hearts with harmony for one another made the greatest improvements. In one weekend, their members had over 102 Reiki students in their classes, far more than had ever attended before.

Through Laurelle's courage and trust in Reiki, she was able to start a process that transformed her Reiki community from one of fear and distrust into one of love and cooperation. By using Reiki to activate the universal law of abundance, not only did her Reiki practice improve, but so did everyone else's. The entire community benefited and Reiki helped many more people than ever before.

Untold benefits wait for any Reiki person who decides to take action and create a more vital, cooperative Reiki community. Reiki is a tremendous power that can help you create a new reality where everyone wins. The universe is always in a state of balance. A problem cannot exist unless the solution exists at the same time. Reiki can help you quickly discover the solution and connect it to the problem to create a wonderful new experience. So do not hesitate to accept any seemingly difficult situation in your Reiki community as an opportunity to demonstrate the healing power of Reiki.

We are moving from a power-and control-centered world into a heart-centered world. Reiki comes from the heart, which is why it is becoming so popular. It is here to help us move into the next phase of human experience, a phase where the truth of the heart will be understood and acted on. Whether people are aware of it or not, we are moving toward a place of honor and respect for each other all over the planet, regardless of the group one belongs to. It is our destiny, and the more we allow it to take place in our own hearts, the faster and easier it will take place for everyone else.

If we as Reiki practitioners are to help this process along, it will be much easier and it makes more sense if we accomplish it within our own community first before attempting to help other groups. The power of Reiki is greatly increased when one is working from a loving, accepting, and empowering Reiki community.

This is the direction the world is moving in and Reiki is here to lead the way. Let's give thanks to be so fortunate to be alive on the planet now and to be able to use Reiki to manifest this great transformation.

Walter, Arjava, and I have gotten to know each other over a number of years. I met Arjava when he invited me to Japan to tour the sacred Reiki sites in Tokyo and Kyoto. I first met Walter in Germany. He invited me to his home after I had taught a Reiki class in the United Kingdom. We had a great time talking about Reiki and hiking at one of the local power spots. Later the three of us met in Japan. We visited Dr. Usui's grave and Mt. Kurama. We had meaningful spiritual experiences together and found that we really enjoy each other's company. We are each from different schools of Reiki, and find the diversity to be stimulating and inspiriting. We are happy we were guided to get to know each other. I have sponsored Arjava's classes here in the United States and also Walter has taught his special Reiki classes at our Reiki Retreat.

We decided to write this book together to share our love and knowledge of Reiki with each other and with the Reiki community. It is our hope that the love that we have for each other and for Reiki will spread to the Reiki community around the world. We hope the love will inspire everyone to take the next step on the spiritual path and continue with greater clarity and purpose. We also hope that people will go against any fear and create meaningful spiritual connections with others. There is no friend like a spiritual friend.

The three of us are also planning to teach a special Reiki workshop together. Once we set it up, we will be teaching it all over the planet.

CHAPTER 23

The Future of Reiki

—by William Lee Rand—

Because of the change that consciousness is undergoing on the planet, Reiki has a wonderful future. Reiki is becoming more popular because of the change, but at the same time it is one of the reasons the change is taking place. In fact, you could say that the spirit of Reiki is the spirit of our planet's future.

The change in consciousness has also been called a paradigm shift. A paradigm shift takes place when the basic assumptions that the world bases its decisions on make a major change.

In the past people have attempted to preserve their well-being by establishing and defending their differences and creating separateness—separateness from other individuals, ethnic groups, religions, countries, etc. Maintaining separateness has been of paramount importance, and groups have devoted the majority of their resources to it. The underlying idea was that peace will come only when we first protect ourselves from others and then dominate them. The result has been weapons of increasingly greater destructiveness and an increasingly less safe world.

The assumption that separateness was the solution to our security came from fear. The fear came mostly from not knowing or understanding members of other groups, religions, countries, etc. Fear creates distortions in ones thinking and this is what caused people to accept this false assumption.

The truth is that we are not separate. We are all interconnected. This principle has been an important part of the teachings of many spiritual groups and native peoples since ancient times. It is also a basic truth of Reiki consciousness. Fortunately, as the world becomes a smaller place and activities in the world have speeded up, the truth has become easier to see. Many of the world's leaders are realizing this and have begun to work more closely together. We can see the evidence in the end of the cold war, the destruction of the Berlin wall, and the fact that the major powers of the world are now working together to solve problems and create peace rather than engaging in or instigating war.

Most of the countries of the world have gotten the message and are beginning to operate under the assumption that if we all work together, everyone will be better off. Although major problems continue in the world, tremendous resources are being focused on them. It appears that we are over the hump. We are quickly moving from a world where separateness, power, and control are the main methods of organization to a world where love, cooperation, and acceptance are becoming the primary basis of our activities. These are the basic qualities that Reiki creates in any person or situation it is directed toward. It is certain that the increased use of Reiki in the world is contributing to this process.

Reiki Will Help Bring World Peace

One of the difficulties the world has experienced is the struggle between different religious and ethnic groups. In fact when we look at the history of the world, we can see that many wars have been fought over religious differences where one religious group try's to dominate the other. Religious conflict has caused great suffering in the world and created religious hatreds that go directly against the most important religious principles. Much of the suffering in the world comes from religious intolerance.

Because Reiki is spiritual, yet not a religion, it has attracted students from all religious and spiritual backgrounds. Catholic priests and nuns practice Reiki. Jews, Protestants, Muslims, Hindus, and Buddhists practice Reiki. Jains, Zoroastrinists, Taoists, and Shintoists practice Reiki. Wiccans, shamans, native peoples, and those on independent spiritual paths practice Reiki. Those in virtually all religious groups are attracted to the practice of Reiki. An important reason is that Reiki gives each person a more immediate experience of the divine. Reiki places everyone more directly in contact with the higher power (regardless of the name one may call it) and provides direct experience of the higher power's grace and compassion. Reiki is thus helping to unite all people of the world regardless of religious or ethnic background.

I notice from traveling all over the world that Reiki people seem to be the same wherever I go. There seems to be a sparkle in the eye and a special positive energy that all Reiki people share. The special energy seems to break through all barriers between those who have Reiki. As more and more people open up to the practice of Reiki, the common thread it provides between all religious groups will help them to see each other as friends rather than enemies.

In addition the fact that Reiki can and is being sent at a distance by many people to heal world crisis situations adds another dimension to the healing Reiki provides. The number of people in the world who practice Reiki will continue to grow, which will increase the help Reiki is providing to create world peace.

Many have experienced the fact that as more people gather together in one group to do Reiki, the strength of each person's Reiki goes up. That's because the total amount of Reiki energy being channeled increases exponentially. If you double the number of people practicing Reiki in a group, rather than having twice as much Reiki flowing, you actually have four times as much. This group dynamic also applies to the number of people in the world practicing Reiki. So as the number of world Reiki practitioners goes up, it causes a tremendous increase in the amount of Reiki flowing in the world. At some point in the near future, a critical point will be reached where there will be so much Reiki flowing on the planet that world peace will come very quickly. In the near future, Reiki, working with all other forms of religious and spiritual practice, will make the difference that brings peace to the world.

When it happens, we will see the members of all religions acknowledging, honoring, and respecting each other. The world's religious leaders will be seen together, working to promote higher spiritual consciousness. In the past, only saints and rare individuals could work miracles and have powerful spiritual experiences. As consciousness shifts into a higher dimension, new possibilities will develop for the "common" person, allowing everyone to have a direct experience of the higher power that produces results in everyday life. Current religions will go through major transformations and new religions will come into being. Reiki will play an important role in these spiritual developments.

The paradigm shift is happening now and the popularity of Reiki is one of the key indicators of this.

In the past Reiki was difficult to explain to others. Often Reiki practitioners would keep their practice to themselves out of fear of ridicule. If Reiki or other healing practices were described on news programs or in the newspaper, it was often done in a derogatory way. Reiki people and other healers were portrayed as being weird and misguided or even worse, as charlatans.

The attitude began to change in the mid-90s. Reiki became more popular and accepted by the general public. News programs began to air short segments on Reiki and portray it in a positive way, often saying "this is what people are doing now" as a way of informing the public of something that is becoming more popular. Scientific research began to be conducted on Reiki with positive results. Alternative medicine in general became more popular. A report by David Eisenburg indicated that in the United States, over 100 million people were receiving some form of alternative health care and spending over 14 billion dollars of their own money for their sessions.

I noticed in the mid-90s that not only were more nurses enrolling in my Reiki classes, but so were some doctors! The doctors and nurses began reporting to me about their experiences practicing Reiki in hospitals and clinics. At first it was difficult and many of their stories were filled with experiences of resistance and difficulty from other members of the hospital staff and the administration. Then as time went by, and Reiki continued to be promoted in hospitals and clinics, the stories began to include more and more successes and greater acceptance of Reiki.

Now at the beginning of the Millennium, Reiki is really gaining a foothold. There are at least 100 hospitals in the United States where Reiki is being offered. In many Reiki has become a regular part of the service the hospital officially offers its patients! In these hospitals, organizations have been started to administer Reiki and other alternative practices. Some have developed protocols, guidelines, and ethics that work in harmony with the hospital and also support the Reiki practitioners and the patients. It is turning into a major success story for Reiki. Some hospitals not offering Reiki want to do so because they notice losing patients to those hospitals with Reiki programs.

The current attitude is so positive for Reiki and other alternative practices in the United States that the trend will certainly grow. I predict that in a short time, Reiki will be offered at most hospitals in the United States. In addition, health insurance programs are now looking at Reiki as a possible insurance benefit. As soon as a few add it, the competitive nature of the health-insurance industry will cause all of them to include Reiki. Then health insurance will pay for Reiki treatments. The need for Reiki practitioners will grow quickly and Reiki will have become established as a normal part of health care in the United States. It will happen easily within the next 10 years!

Looking further into the future, I see advances made in the effectiveness of Reiki treatments. As science gets involved in studying what makes Reiki work, the increased understanding will be used to improve its effectiveness. Also, as more and more people practice Reiki and continue to heal the deeper aspects of themselves, improvements will be made and they will become better healers. With all this attention from both the spiritual and the scientific communities, breakthroughs are bound to happen, creating even greater benefits. I see no end to the process of improvement. In the future, when a person gets sick, many hospitals will use Reiki first to heal the patient, and in most cases, because of the improved effectiveness, Reiki will be all the patient will need. Only if Reiki does not heal the patient would the doctor consider using allopathic methods.

The spiritual nature of Reiki will continue to develop also. We have seen that new forms of Reiki are continually being channeled. Some of these are more powerful. People are having more meaningful spiritual experiences from their attunements and treatments. The validation of Reiki by science and its complete acceptance by the public will move Reiki into a position of great importance. The increased use of Reiki by more and more people and its examination from different perspectives will quicken the process of development. Attunements and treatments will become increasingly more effective.

The higher power is infinite in nature, so no limit exists to what can come from it. As we surrender more completely to the power of Reiki, the superconscious mind from which Reiki comes will be able to heal us more and more deeply. As this happens, we will become better able to hold and ground higher consciousness within our physical bodies. Our awareness will expand. We will channel ever-higher qualities of Reiki energy, which will produce even more meaningful healing. So strong will this energy become, that eventually the veils of illusion that prevent us from knowing our true nature will be dissolved and released. At first a few, but then quickly more, people will enter satori and become self-realized. The higher state of mind, which only a very few people on earth have experienced, will become the normal state for everyone. Our mission as a race of people will have been completed. The peace, love, and freedom of the higher power will be established as the predominant power on the planet. Reiki will have fulfilled its divine purpose on earth.

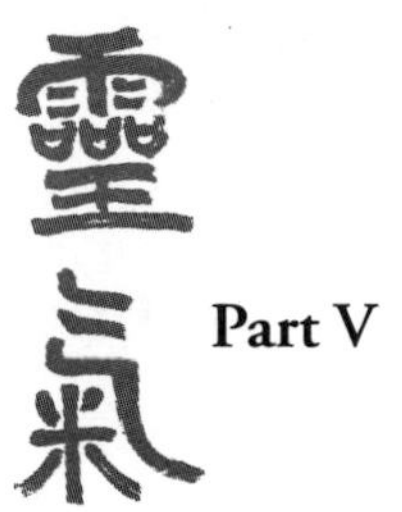

Part V

APPENDIX

CHAPTER 24

Pronunciation Guide for All Japanese and Other Foreign Words

—by Frank Arjava Petter—

Akimoto, Shizuko	= *ah-kee-mo-to, she-zoo-ko*	
Amaterasu	= *ama-teh-la-sue*	
Arjava	= *r-java (as in the letter R, and coffee)*	
Bi	= *be*	美
Butcho	= *boot-cho*	
Byogen	= *bjo-gen*	病原
Byosen	= *bjo-sen*	病腺
Chikara	= *chi-kah-la*	力
Chiryo	= *chi-lee-oh*	治療
Dainichi Nyorai	= *die-knee-chi, njo-lie*	
Do	= *doe*	働
Doi, Hiroshi	= *doe-eeh, he-roe-she*	
Doshisha	= *dough-she-shah ("dough" as in doughnuts, "shah" as in the Shah of Persia)*	
En	= *en*	縁
Enkaku	= *en-kakoo*	遠隔
Gakkai	= *guck-kai ("guck" as in muck, "kai" as in hi)*	
Gassho	= *gush-show*	
Gedoku	= *geh-dre-ku*	下毒
Genetsu	= *gen-net-tzu*	下熱

Gifu	= *ghee-foo ("ghee" as in Indian clarified butter, "foo" as in fool)*	
Go-to	= *go-toe*	
Goto, Shinpei	= *go-toe, shin-pay*	
Gyoshi	= *gyo-sche*	凝視
Hanshin	= *hun-shin*	半身
Hanshin ko ketsu-Ho	= *hun-schin-koe-cat-sue-hoe*	半身交血法
Hayashi, Chujiro	= *ha-ya-she, chu-gee-low*	
Hesso	= *heh-sso*	臍
Hibiki	= *he-be-key*	
Hikkei	= *he-kay*	
Ho	= *hoe*	法
Jacki kiri joka-ho	= *jacki-keeri joker-hoe*	
Joshin Kokyuu-Ho	= *joe-shin-koh-kjue-hoe*	浄心呼吸法
Kakaricho	= *ka-ka-lee-cho*	
Kanji	= *cun-gee*	
Katcho	= *cut-cho*	
Katsugen Undo	= *cut-tzu-gen oon-doe*	
Ken	= *ken*	健
Kenyoku	= *ken-yo-koo*	乾浴
Kobayashi, Chetna	= *co-bah-ya-she, chat-na*	
Kobe	= *ko-bay*	

Kohai	= *ko-hi*	
Koki	= *koe-key*	呼気
Kokoro	= *koe-koe-low*	心
Kondo	= *con-do (as in condominium)*	
Koyama	= *co-yama*	
Kurama	= *koo-lama ("koo" as in cool, "lama" as in Tibetan monk)*	
Koto	= *kyoe-toe*	
Latihan	= *la-tea-hun*	
Makoto	= *ma-koe-toe*	誠
Mawashi	= *ma-wa-she*	回し
Meiji	= *may-jee*	
Mochizuki, Toshitaka	= *mae-chi-zoo-key, toe-she-tah-kah*	
Meiso	= *may-so*	
Nasruddin, Mullah	= *nus-rue-deen, moo-lah*	
Noguchi (Haruchika)	= *no-goo-chi, ha-loo-chi-kah*	
Ogawa	= *oh-ga-wa*	
Oishi	= *o-ee-she*	
Okuden	= *o-koo-den*	
Osho	= *o-show*	
Reiji	= *ley-ghee*	霊
Reiju	= *ley-jew*	
Reiki	= *ley-key*	靈氣
Roku-to	= *lock-ooh-toe*	
Ryoho	= *lee-oh-hoe*	
Sadako	= *sadah-koh*	
Sai	= *sigh*	才
Saihoji	= *sigh-hoe-gee ("sigh" as in sigh, "hoe" as in garden tool, "g" as in the letter G)*	
San-to	= *sun-toe*	
satori	= *sat-oh-ree ("sat" as in Saturday, "oh" as in oh, "lee" as in jeans)*	

Seiheki chiryo	= *say-heh-key chi-lee-oh*	性癖治療
Seitai	= *say-thai*	
Senpai	= *sen-pie*	
Sensei	= *sen-say*	
Shacho	= *sha-cho*	
Shashin chiryo	= *sha-shin, chi-lee-oh*	写真治療
Shihan	= *she-hun*	
Shihan Kaku	= *she-hun, kah-koo*	
Shinpeden	= *shin-pee-den*	
Shinto	= *shin-toe*	
Shizuoka	= *she-zoo-oh-ka(r)*	
Shoden	= *show-den*	
Shu Chu	= *shoe-chu (as in choose)*	
Subud	= *sue-bood*	
Takata, Hawayo	= *t-a kah-tah, ha-wah-yo*	
Taketomi	= *takeh-toe-me*	
Tai	= *thai (as in Thailand)*	体
Taireidou	= *thai-ley-doe*	
Tanden	= *tun-den*	丹田
Taniai	= *tah-knee-i*	
Tenno	= *ten-noe*	
Tokyo	= *toe-kyoe*	
Tsutome	= *tzu-toe-meh*	
Uchi	= *oo-chi*	
Undo	= *oon-doe*	
Ushida	= *oo-she-da*	
Usui, Mikao	= oo-su-ey, *me-kah-oh ("kah" as in card with a longer "a")*	
Waka	= *wah-kah*	

Wanabe	= *wah-na-bay*
Watanabe	= *wah-tah-na-bay*
Yago	= *yah-go ("yah" as in yahoo, "go" as in leave)*
Yamagata	= *yama-gutta ("yama" as in yard, "gutta" as in gut-a)*
Yon-to	= *yohn-toe*
Zenki	= *zen-key*

CHAPTER 25

Conduct in Japan and at Japanese Reiki Sites

—by Frank Arjava Petter—

For those of you who are determined to visit the Reiki sites in Japan, I would like to share a few guidelines on how to behave. As foreigners in Japan, we are not expected to know proper etiquette—after all, we are just foreigners.

To illustrate my point, here is a little story about a British friend of mine. Rob had been in Japan several times and was talking to a foreign friend at a bar. They had already consumed a few beers when the friend suddenly said, "I bet you a hundred bucks that you won't go into a *Sento* (Japanese public bath) wearing a gorilla suit."

This isn't something Rob needed to hear twice. He got a gorilla suit and went into the public bath. Once there, he expected to be kicked out or to have people stare and laugh at him, insult him, beat him up, invite him for a drink, or ask him to perform at a kid's party—or all of the above.

He squeezed the gorilla's head under his arm and proceeded to take a shower, soaping his hairy gorilla's back and neck and enjoying himself immensely. What he did not expect was the total lack of a reaction in the overcrowded bath. No one took any notice of him, except for a small boy who said, "Daddy, I'm scared." Without giving it a second thought, his father replied, "Don't worry, son. It's just a foreigner"

Although foreigners aren't expected to know etiquette, if you behave well in Japan, people will be willing to talk to you and open up. Before discussing some of the rituals that people perform when entering a temple or approaching a grave, I'd like to include a list of what **not** to do in Japan:

- Don't hug and kiss in public, especially not in the presence of someone you respect. Holding hands is permitted but frowned upon.

Several years ago, we took a couple of German friends to a museum depicting the life of the *Ainu* (the native people of Hokkaido). When the two of them kissed in public, a Japanese lady yelled, "This is Japan!" Because she naturally yelled in Japanese, they didn't understand. It may occasionally be useful not to understand the language in Japan (a strategy I sometimes use), but don't try to change Japanese culture by force!

- Don't argue with Japanese officials unless your Japanese is superb. Losing your temper is seen as a loss of face. Most likely, the official will become absolutely immovable, and your request will be turned down without further consideration. Once you have been turned down, a "repentant" letter may mend the situation. But be sure to have such a letter written by a Japanese national.
- Don't drink and drive. Not even one alcoholic drink is permitted when you operate a motor vehicle.
- Stay away from drugs. The Japanese punishment for drug abuse is severe. Foreign offenders are a welcome feast for the authorities.
- Stay away from cabaret shows, unless a Japanese business associate invites you there.
- Stay away from gangs. The movie *Black Rain* did not exaggerate with regard to motorcycle gangs.
- Don't wear shoes inside a Japanese house or in the *tatami* (straw-mat) room of a restaurant.
- Don't accept an invitation from Japanese people unless you are absolutely sure they really mean it. In many cases, an invitation is offered out of politeness. To be invited to a private home is a very rare occurrence and considered to be a great honor.
- Don't believe that a smile equals a "yes." Japanese people often feel they would hurt someone's feelings by saying "no." A smile will sometimes mean either "no," "I am sorry," "I don't know," "forget it," or "leave me alone!"

When visiting a temple or shrine:

- Generally wear clean clothing and be polite. Don't talk too loudly or run around. Turn off your cell phone. Don't take photographs of people without asking them first. Don't enter roped-off areas. Before entering the main gate, fold your hands in front of your heart in the *gassho* position and bow once toward the temple.

Many shrines and temples have either holy springs or at least a fountain at their main entrance. You should purify yourself here in the following manner:

- Take the (usually) wooden or bamboo ladle and draw some water with it. Clean the ladle. Then fill it again and pour the water over your free hand. Then take the ladle in the other hand and clean your second hand.
- If there is a statue at the springs (like the one at the entrance of Kurama Temple), fill the ladle and clean the statue by gently splashing some water on it. If the water is drinking water (you must inquire about this beforehand), you can also rinse out your mouth. (This ritual is not necessarily performed by each Japanese person who enters a shrine or temple.) Now enter the temple grounds.

At a Japanese graveyard:

- Wear clean clothing and behave as you would when visiting your own relative's grave. Bring flowers and incense, several candles, a lighter/matches, and a small garbage bag.
- When you enter the graveyard at Saihoji, on your right side you will find a small hut that houses a water pump and pile of pails and ladles. Take a pail and ladle with you, first filling the pail with fresh water.
- Go to the grave and clean off any debris on it, including leaves and twigs. Remove any old withered flowers left on the grave, and replace them with the fresh ones you have brought. Japanese graves usually have built-in vases.
- Once the grave site is clean, take the pail of water and ladle and wash the grave marker, the pathway that leads to the grave, and the memorial stone, if necessary. (You may have to return to the pump and refill the pail several times.). If the person buried there liked Japanese sake (rice wine), you can also wash the grave marker with rice wine. But don't climb all over the grave in the process.
- After you have cleaned the grave and put the flowers in the vase, you can place the incense in the incense holder. Then place your candles on the grave and light them. Take a step back, fold your hands in front of your heart, and say a prayer.
- It is acceptable to take photographs at Japanese graves. Everybody does it. In fact, it is a Japanese tradition to take photos at the grave of a loved one. I have taken twelve sets of pictures of my parents-in-law in front of their family grave—one set for every year!

CHAPTER 26

The Meiji Emperor's Poems

—by Frank Arjava Petter together with Chetna Kobayashi—

The 125 Meiji Emperor's poems, called *gyosei,* are written in the so-called waka form. The waka consists of five syllables in the first line, seven syllables in the second, five syllables in the third, seven syllables in the fourth, and seven syllables in the fifth line. Dr. Usui used them in his Reiki meetings to help his students focus their attention on what is essential.

The poems were written by the Meiji emperor (who ruled Japan from 1868–1912) in ancient Japanese and my mother in law, Masano Kobayashi, translated them into contemporary Japanese before my wife Chetna and I translated them into English. My comments are set in parenthesis. At times I changed the sequence of the lines to make them more easily understood in English.

Each poem has a headline.

The first fourteen poems were already translated and published in my second book, *Reiki—The Legacy of Dr. Usui.*

On pages 12, 42, 100 and 244 you can find four poems written in Japanese calligraphy.

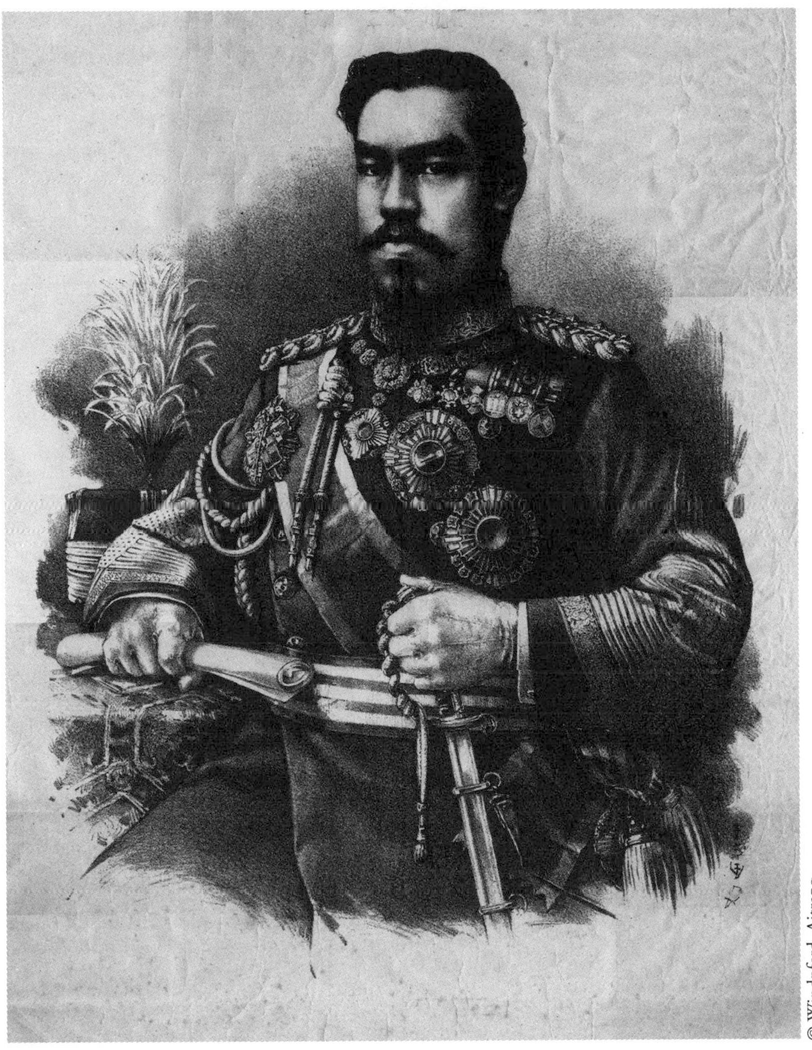

The Meiji-Emperor

: 1—*The Moon*
Profound change occurs
Because so many people
Have gone from this world
But the moon in an autumn
Night
Remains (always) the same

: 2—*The Sky*
Light green* and cloudless
The big sky
I too would like to have
Such a spirit (kokoro)

: 3—*In General*
Whenever I think
Of the farmers suffering from the heat
In the rice paddies
I can not say it is hot
Even if this is the case

: 4—*The Wind of Falling Leaves*
It takes so much rain
To give the perfect color
To the maple leaves
But they are blown away
By a single gust of wind

: 5—*In General*
Understand (life) by
Seeing how the stone has
Been
Hollowed out by rain
Don't cling to the illusion
That nothing changes

* The word light-green is always used in connection with the sky in poetry. In Japanese, there is a different concept of the colors "green" and "blue." The traffic signal that we call "green" is considered to be "blue" in Japan. However, the color is the same!

: 6—*In General*
I do not need
To be angry at the heavens
Or put the blame on
Others (for my suffering)
If I see my own faults

: 7—*In General*
There is so much
blame in this world
So do not worry
About it too much

: 8—*Friend(ship)*
Being friends
Being able to show
Each other our errors
Is the true shrine
Of friendship

: 9—*A Pine Tree on a Rock*
Stormy world
Human mind (kokoro)
Remain as still
As the pine tree
Rooted on a rock

: 10—*The Wave*
One moment stormy
The next it is calm
The wave in the ocean
Is actually
Just like the human existence

: 11—*In General*
If the background
You come from is wealthy
And without personal problems
Your human obligations
Are easily forgotten

: 12—*Siblings*
Sometimes in this world
The wind shakes the house
But troubles are overcome
If the branches (siblings) of
The tree (family)
Grow up harmoniously

: 13—*The Spirit* (Kokoro)
Whatever happens
In any situation
It is my wish that
The spirit (kokoro) remains
Without boundaries (free)

: 14—*Medicine*
Instead of buying
A great deal of medicine
It is better to take care
Of your (own) body

: 15—*In General*
At night
The sound of the mosquitoes
Makes me wonder
What bank of the river
And in what field
The ones who went to war
Had to spend the night on

: 16—*Education*
Young (Japanese) ladies
Study hard
And think of (all) virtuous people
As of your teachers

: 17—*Fallen Flowers on the Water*
What is most enjoyable
About the flowers
Blossoming by the pond
They still float on the water
After they fall
And you can see their beautiful shape

: 18—*The Firefly in Front of the Moon*
Accommodating the moon's
Reflection in the pond
The humbleness of the firefly
Hiding-
Behind the stalks of a reed

: 19—*A Gemstone**
The most beautiful gemstone
Without the tiniest flaw
May loose its luster
Due to a tiny fleck of dust
If you don't take care of it

: 20—*In General*
Studying children:
Don't compete with one another
Instead—
Take one step
At a time

: 21—*Obedience, Duty* (toward ones parents)
Even though you live
In a (very) busy world
Don't forget
To take care
Of your own parents

: 22—*Grass*
Though the grass
Doesn't look too promising
You may find medicinal herbs (in its midst)
If you look
Carefully

* Maybe he is talking about his position as emperor.

: 23—(To) ***Graduating Students***

Graduated children:
You might think
That you finally made it
But there is no end
To learning

: 24—*The Fringed Pink*

When I seeded, I thought
It was all the same kind of seed
But (now) it blossoms
With a variety of flowers
The Fringed Pink

: 25—*Waterfall*

A rock obstructing the river
Increases the sound of the waterfall
That you can't hear
The sound of running water
Or any other sound

: 26—*Water*

Water is flexible enough
To fit any vessel
Still it has the power
To go through rock

: 27—*Grass*

Shameful mole
Worked his way underground
And all the roots
Of what you have planted
Died

: 28—*Old Man*

The old man
Who came out to welcome me
Supported by his grandchild
Is now standing up
On his own

: 29—*A Tree Covered with Mud**

When I see
Trees covered with mud
It reminds me
That there must be people
Who live in obscurity

: 30—*A Visitor in the Snow*

Old man:
Coming (to greet me)
Without waiting
For the snow to subside
Please come closer to the fire

: 31—*Calligraphy*

Whether a character
Is written beautifully
Or not
A letter
Should be easy to read

: 32—*Parents*

The spirit of parenthood:
Even though
You grow old
Your parents still think of you
As a child

: 33—*In General*

Soldiers who go to war
Leave the old folks at home
How courageous
And dedicated
(They are) for their country!

* Mud slides are common in the rainy season in Japan. The emperor must be talking here about the old caste system.

: 34—*Bird(s)*
The birds flying freely
In the big sky
Won't forget
Their home
To return to

: 35—*Learning*
You should know
From the way
The children learn
When you practice more
You (will) get better results

: 36—*Dewdrops on the Fringed Pink*
Young female students
Gathering on campus
Look as fresh
As if they were Fringed Pinks
(Adorned) with dewdrops

: 37—*Sincerity*
The sincerity
Of the human heart
In this world
Makes even a wrathful deity
Cry

: 38—*In General*
It is appropriate
To enjoy the flowers
After completing the work
You are supposed to do

: 39—*Reminiscence*
People don't look
At themselves
And talk only
About the others
That's what society is (all about)

: 40—*Mountain Peak*
Scraping the big sky
The mountain seems so high
But if you don't give up
And set out to conquer (it)
There will be a path.

: 41—*In General*
You should talk
To others
Only
After you have made up
Your (own) mind

: 42—*In General*
If whatever you think
Comes true
Don't let it get to your head
And don't
Forget to be humble

: 43—*In General*
So many things to do
(And) so much to think (about)
What you can do
However
Is limited

: 44—*A Pine Tree in the Snow*
(When) the snow is piling up
On the weak branch
Of a pine tree
Come closer
And sweep it off

: 45—*In General*
Those who died in the war
For their country
To last forever
Let me record their names
For the future

: 46—*The Fan*
Even in the daytime heat
People come (to see me)
Let me turn on the fan
For them

: 47—*Spirit*
It is rather beautiful
In its simplicity
When you are
Concerned
With the spirit (kokoro)

: 48—*Reminicence*
Keep making an effort
When it seems difficult
It is possible
To achieve anything
In this world

: 49—*A Pillar*
One
Who is the pillar
Of the family
Shouldn't (need to) mind
Small things

: 50—*Reminiscing about Grass*
(Be careful!)
You may have said something
Without deeper thoughts
And this may take root
In society

: 51—*Reminiscing about Boats*
It is easy to go down (stream)
On a river boat
The world is like that
Don't neglect to pay attention
To the rudder

: 52—*Reminiscing about Gemstones*
Everyone in society says
This gemstone
Is so wonderful
But there are very few
Which (in fact) are flawless

: 53—*The Feeling during Travels*
Each time
I go on a trip
I wonder if I am
Disturbing
(My own) people's life

: 54—*Humanity*
For (your) own country
You beat the enemy
But don't forget
The issues (at home)
You really need to care
About

: 55—*Medicine*
For (the good of our) country
I would like
To give the elixir of immortality
To the old man
Whom I would like to live on

: 56—*Old Folks (the Elderly)*
The elderly
Repeat their memories
Over and over
But hidden in their words
Are valuable teachings

: 57—*Evening*
When the sun
Begins to set
I miss the day
That I spent
Idle

: 58—*The Parents Heart*
The spring night dream
Of the pheasants
Who worry about their offspring
In the burned field, I guess
Won't be peaceful

: 59—*Medicine*
Advice from
The sincere
Is like useful medicine
Even
To the healthy

: 60—*In General*
Even a busy man
Can make time
For whatever
He really wants
To do

: 61—*Summer Grass*
The summer grass
Represents
The busy world
It keeps coming up
Though you keep cutting it down

: 62—*Mind*
When the mind is relaxed
Without any obstacle
There is more danger
Than when you have
An enemy around you

: 63—*The Narrow Path*
The narrow path between
Countryside rice paddies
Is really tiny but the villagers
Give way to one another
And use the space
Thoughtfully

: 64—*A Rice Paddy House**
The young ones gone to war
An old man alone
Taking care
Of rice paddies
In the mountain

: 65—*A Day*
I would like
My spirit
Rejuvenated
Just like
The rising sun

: 66—*Monsoon Season*
Because
Of the monsoon
The surface of the straw mats (tatami)
Gets so moist and wet
I worry about the villagers' homes

: 67—*A Thought in a Cold Night*
Cold night
Awoke from a dream
By the sound of the storm
And I worry
About the houses of the villagers

: 68—*A Precious Gemstone*
The precious stone
Is not shining
It seems
Because you forgot
To polish it

---

* We are not sure whether the emperor may have made this word up himself—it is not in the dictionary.

: 69—*The Clock*
Some of them go faster
And some of them slower
All clocks
Have different sizes
And different hands

: 70—*The Road**
It would be better
Not to take the dangerous road
Even though
You might think
You'll get there faster

: 71—*In General*
You must consider
The timing
When to proceed or not
Otherwise you may step
Onto a dangerous path

: 72—*The Heart*
The childhood's heart:
Too bad
One day we forget
Our own innocence
Completely

: 73—*The Child*
I wish the young bamboo
In the garden to grow up straight
But it readily
Leans over
In many directions

* The Japanese word "michi" stands for "way" in terms of Tao.

: 74—*Blossom That Looks Like a Cloud*
Mountain cherry trees
In (full) blossom
Cloud-like
In between
Stunted pine trees

: 75—*Houses in the Summer*
Right next to each other
Houses in town
Must be very hot
Through the narrow windows
The wind can't get in

: 76—*Devotion for One's Parents*
Caring for
One's own parents with love
Is the beginning
Of the human being's
Sincerity

: 77—*The Parent's Heart*
Anybody will
Remember and understand
The parent's heart
When they age
Themselves

: 78—*Suggestion, Advice*
The teaching of the parents
Consists of tiny things
But still it is the base for you
To go (and take)
Into the spacious world

: 79—*The Word and Feeling for Flowers*
Even though they fall right after they open
Mountain cherry blossoms
Flower and spread their fragrance
For years and years
Without ever complaining

: 80—*Dust*
It is good
To get rid of the dust
When it accumulates
Even though you may not find
Anything wonderful underneath it

: 81—*Learning*
I regret
My childhood attitude
That learning is
Not worth
The effort

: 82—*Reminiscense*
I think about
(My) people's life
How they live
Come rain
Come shine

: 83—*A Road*
(The goal) far off
But if you take the path
The human should travel (upon)
I suppose
There won't be any danger

: 84—*In General*
Time flies
Like an arrow
You should work
Swiftly
Whatever you do

: 85—*A Boat in between the Reeds*
Be patient
With the oar
The little boat in the reeds
Can't move
Freely

: 86—*Road*
Studying, you may need
To take a break
And start again
Because the path of learning
Is not an easy one

: 87—*In General*
To reach
The end of your life
Without accomplishment
It is not worth
Living long in the world

: 88—*People, Human*
Things may not seem to work out
As you wish
But they turn out to be good
When you look back
At your (own) life

: 89—*Mind*
On a day
When wind and surf
Are quiet
The captain of the boat
Will be extra careful

: 90—*The Road*
If your are slower
Than the others
You are walking with
You must (still)
Take the right path

: 91—*In General*
So many dewdrops
On the Fringed Pinks
Without shaking them off
They may bend
In an unforeseeable direction

: 92—*A Gemstone**
A gemstone
Chosen by so many
Out of so many stones
Still one or the other blemish remains
That's the nature of this world

: 93—*The Parent's Heart*
When parents
Look at their own children
They think of them as tiny
Even though they're grown and independent
Such is the nature of parenthood

: 94—*Parents*
Don't forget
What your parents
Have given to you
Even though you think
You are on your own

: 95—*Mine*
If there were
A mountain of gold, radiating
How can you
See the light
Without opening

* The emperor about himself.

: 96—*In General*
When you enter
A wide and spacious road
You should be careful
The world is
Full of stumbling blocks

: 97—*Reminiscence*
Involved
In extraordinary work
In the big world
One must be concerned
With uncountable details

: 98—*Mind*
Wide and spacious world
Communicating
The human mind
Easily gets trapped
In (its own) narrow spaces

: 99—*Old Folks*
You should not complain
Just because
You have grown old
There is a (graceful) way
To live with old age

: 100—*Home Owner* (the Head of the Family)
The family prospers
If the head of the family
Is as grounded
As the main pole of the house

: 101—*Reminiscing*
Leading the country
For it to be looked upon
As good
I do my best
Using my abilities
To the maximum*

* Literally: using my head as hundreds of heads.

: 102—*Teacher*
Even if you become a specialist
Of some subject
Don't forget
What was given to you
By your teachers

: 103—*The Newspaper*
So many people read the paper
Therefore
One should write
About the meaningful
Instead of the mundane

: 104—*Water*
Too bad
Though the source
Is pure and clear
Water becomes soiled
When it flows into a polluted stream

: 105—*Cows*
The cow doesn't stumble
Because there is no hurry
No matter
If the cart is heavier
Than she can pull

: 106—*The God of Sky and Earth*
The one who is not shy
Toward the invisible
God
Has found the truth
In his heart

: 107—*In General*
Don't complain about
Things not moving along
Smoothly
But look
At your own laziness

: 108—*Friends*
The most useful strength
Of this world
Is close friendship
To help each other with

: 109—*Old Pine Tree*
Thousand-year-old pine tree
In the garden
I would like to help you
Live longer and longer
With all my good care

: 110—*The Farmers*
The villagers tending to
The rice paddies in the mountains
Won't have peace and quiet
From seeding
To harvest time

: 111—*The Pine Tree*
The pine tree
That grew
With patience
Through storm and snowfall
Looks more valuable (to me)

: 112—*The Country*
Keep up the good
And drop the bad
Let's make this country
Equally good
To the other countries

: 113—*In General*
Even though
Very famous
In this world
One should be humble
As a human being

: 114—*The Snail*
What is going on
Out there
That is how a snail
Comes out of its house
To take a look

: 115—*The Road*
If you are walking
On the right path
No danger
Of this world
Will affect you

: 116—*The Treasure*
Work hard
Accomplish a skill
And become independent in the world
This way the skill
Becomes your treasure

: 117—*Students*
Even though the world
Is not quiet, but noisy
The student should not stray
From the path of learning
With a quiet heart

: 118—*In General*
When required
To walk forward
Go ahead, otherwise
You will reach after
The others in this world

: 119—(*Spiritual*) *Practice*
Chosen to be
A leader
Of the world
One must have
The right attitude

: 120—(Spiritual) *Practice*
Unless your work points
Toward the higher good*
It is very hard
To lead
The people in this world

: 121—*Statement of the Right Way of Thinking*
Across the ocean
And in all directions
I am thinking
Of all people as brothers
What is the point of war in this world

: 122—*In General*
Laying there:
A Fringed Pink
Brought to the river bank
By the current
Still blossoming. . .

: 123—(*Children's*) *Play*
Even though you find a game
You would like to play
Don't neglect
The important things
In life

: 124—*In General*
Look at yourself
Often,
Unknowingly
You might get lost
And make mistakes

: 125—*The Mirror*
I should polish my self
More and more
To use the others' clear
And shining heart
As a mirror

* wordly: aim to the general welfare.

About the Authors:

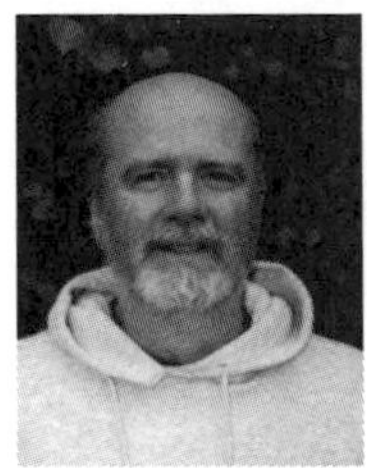

William Lee Rand

William Lee Rand has lived in Hawaii, California, and Michigan. He has a broad background in metaphysics, including twenty years of experience as a hypnotherapist. William has specialized in past-life-regression therapy and spiritual development and is certified in Neuro-Linguistic Programming by the *Robbins Research Institute* in California. While living in Hawaii, he worked with a Kahuna healer. William has also gone to both the North and South Poles to place specially prepared World Peace Crystal Grids to promote world peace. He is founder of *The International Center for Reiki Training* in Southfield, Michigan and is the publisher of the *Reiki News.* He has also written *Reiki—The Healing Touch* and *Reiki for a New Millennium* along with over forty articles on Reiki, and has recorded and produced seven audio tapes. In 1981 William took First Degree Reiki from Bethal Phaigh on the Big Island of Hawaii. Bethal was one of Takata's original Masters. In 1982 he took Second Degree Reiki from Bethal. William has received the master training from four Reiki masters and has taken Reiki training from many others. Since 1989 he has been teaching and giving Reiki seminars worldwide. Always seeking to learn more, his research into Reiki is an ongoing process. William teaches Reiki full time in classes worldwide. (Contact address: www.reiki.org)

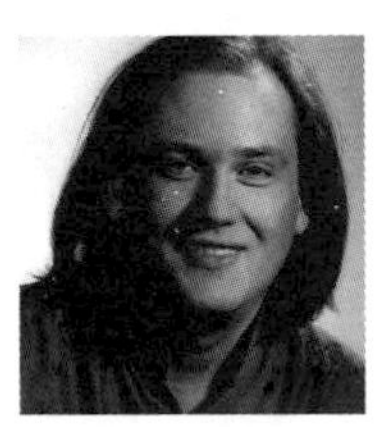

Walter Lübeck

Walter Lübeck (Aquarius, Asc. Sagittarius) has been active as a spiritual teacher since 1988. Throughout the world, he teaches the Rainbow Reiki System that he has developed, Three-Rays Meditation, and Lemurian Tantra in both the German and English languages. The three principles of personal responsibility, love, and consciousness are an important guideline for him in his private and professional life. With his work, he would like to contribute to the dawning of a new golden age on Earth as soon as possible. He has made the results of his research available to the public in 20 books (6 of which on the topic of Reiki) that have been translated into more than a dozen languages, diverse articles in specialized magazines, and teaching videos. He finds it very important for spiritual knowledge to be used for increasing the holistic quality of life. With his diversified training in Reiki, meditation, NLP, shamanism, tantra, homeopathy, nutrition, inner martial arts, feng shui, and work with crystals, he attempts to unite the various esoteric paths and their knowledge in order to optimally help his students progress on their individual paths. An enthusiastic musician, he likes to use drums, didgeridoo, voice, and dance in rituals and spiritual healing. (Contact address: www.rainbowreiki.de)

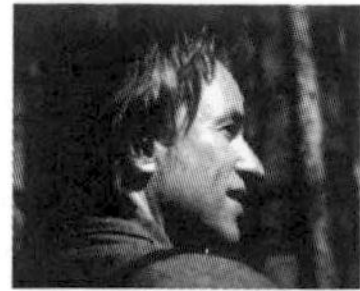

Frank Arjava Petter

In 1993 he brought Reiki back to the land of its origin and was the first Westener to teach the Reiki Master/Teacher Degree in Japan. Together with his Japanese wife, Chetna, he traced back the various Reiki streams to their roots, the original system of Dr. Mikao Usui. He discovered, along with exciting historical facts, fascinating healing techniques new to the West.

Frank Arjava Petter currently teaches together with his wife, Chetna, original Reiki techniques worldwide, in seminars and lectures. His books *Reiki Fire, Reiki—The Legacy of Dr. Usui* and *The Original Reiki Handbook of Dr. Mikao Usui* have already become international bestsellers. (Contact address: www.reikidharma.com)

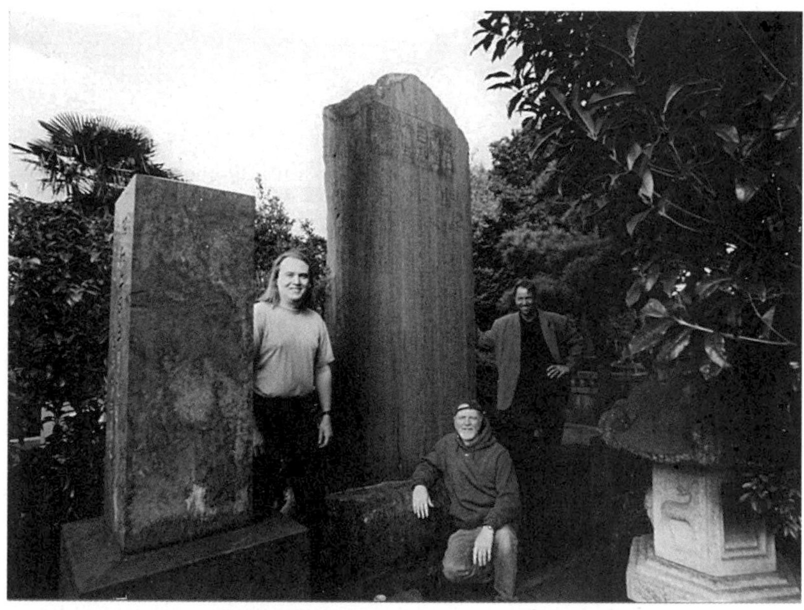

Walter, Frank Arjava and William Lee visiting Usui's memorial stone

Notes

1) Inscription on Usui Memorial, Saihoji Temple, Suginami, Tokyo, Japan. Published in "Reiki Fire" by Frank Arjava Petter, Lotus Light · Shangri-La, Twin Lakes, WI, 1997, third edition, "Dr Usui's Memorial Inscription" on page 28 ff.

2) The information comes from Tatsumi-san, one of Dr. Hayashi's last students, who was interviewed by Melissa Riggall in the summer of 1996.

3) Iyashi No Te: "Healing Hands" by Toshitaka Mochizuki (Japanese edition).

4) "Searching the Roots of Reiki," by Shiomi Takai, published in the magazine *The Twilight Zone*, April 1986, pages 140–143. The article can be viewed on the Web at http://www.pwpm.com/threshold/origins2.html. Note that the Japanese magazine is out of business.

5) *Encyclopedia Britannica*. The 1997 CD-ROM article entitled, "Earthquakes Tokyo-Yokohama. "

6) Dr. Usui: "The Reiki Ryoho Handbook" (English: "The Original Reiki Handbook of Dr. Mikao Usui" by Dr. Mikao Usui and Frank Arjava Petter, Lotus Press · Shangri-La Twin Lakes, WI, 1999, second edition.)

7) Hawayo Takata's Reiki certificate, a copy of which can be obtained from the International Center for Reiki Training. Information also taken from Hawayo Takata's handwritten notes dated May 1936.

8) Petter, F. A. : "Reiki —The Legacy of Dr. Usui", Lotus Press · Shangri-La, Twin Lakes, WI, 1998.

9) Doi Hiroshi: "Iyashi no Gendai Reiki Ho" (ISBN 4-906631-34-7.)

10) Quoted according to Chong-Sok Choe's "Qi, ein religioeses Urwort in China" ("Qi, A Religious Primal Word in China"), Peter Lang Europaeischer Verlag der Wissenschaften.

11) More information on this can be found in the chapter on Reiki Essences in Walter Lübeck's book *Rainbow Reiki*, released by Lotus Light· Shangri-La, Twin Lakes, WI, 1997.

12) Bouligand, Y.: "Liquid Crystals and Their Analogs in Biological Systems." In: Liebert, L. (ed.) *Liquid Crystals. Solid State Physics.* Supplement 14/1978, pages 259-294.

13) Becker, R.O.: "Evidence for a Primitive DC Electrical Analog System Controlling Brain Function." In: *Subtle Energies* 2(1)/1991, pages 71-88.

14) Cohen D., Edelsack E. A., Zimmerman J.E.: "Magnetocardiograms Taken inside a Shielded Room with a Superconducting Point-Contact Magnetometer." In: *Applied Physics Letter* 16/1970, pages 278-280.

15) Smith C.W.: "Biological Effects of Weak Electromagnetic Fields." In: Ho M.W., Popp F-A., Warnke U. (eds) *Bioelectrodynamics and Biocommunication.* World Scientific, Singapore, 1994, ch. 3, pages 81-107.

16) Seto A., Kusaka C., Nakazato S. et al: "Detection of Extraordinary Large Biomagnetic Field Strength from Human Hand." In: *Acupuncture and ElectroTherapeutics Research International Journal,* 1992, pages 17,75-94.

17) Andersen P., Andersson S.A.: "Physiological Basis of the Alpha Rhythm." Appleton-Century Crofts, New York, 1968.

18) Fröhlich H.: "Coherent Electric Vibrations in Biological Systems and the Cancer Problem." *IEEE Transactions on Microwave Theory and Techniques MTT,* 26/1978, pages: 613-617.

19) Sisken B.F., Walker J.: "Therapeutic Aspects of Electromagnetic Fields for Soft-Tissue Healing." In: Blank M. (ed.) *Electromagnetic Fields: Biological Interactions and Mechanisms. Advances in Chemistry Series 250.* American Chemical Society, Washington DC, 1995, pages 277-285.

20) Rein G.: "Biological Effects of Quantum Fields and Their Role in the Natural Healing Process." In: *Frontier Perspectives* 7(1)/1998, pages 16-23.

21) Oshmann, J.: "Energy, Medicine—The Scientific Basis", Churchill Livingstone, Edinburgh 2000, page 206.

22) Cohen Kenneth S.: "The Way of Qigong—The Art and Science of Chinese Energy Healing", Ballantine Books, 1999, ISBN: 0345421094.

23) Namikoshi Toru: "The Complete Book of Shiatsu Therapy", Japan Pubns., 1994, ISBN: 087040461X.

24) You can find these instructions on William Lee Rand's website (www.reiki.org) or on Frank Arjava and Chetna's website (www.reikidharma.com).

25) Hall, Edward T./Hall, Mildreed Reed: "Hidden Differences", Anchor Books, Doubleday.

26) Information on books by Haruchika Noguchi at Zenzei Publishing Company, Tokyo, Japan.

27) Also see Walter Lübeck: "Reiki for First Aid", Lotus Light · Shangri-La, Twin Lakes, WI, 1995.

28) A very extensive list of special positions can be found in Walter Lübeck's book "The Complete Reiki Handbook" Lotus Light · Shangri-La, Twin Lakes, WI 1994, 5th edition. An abbreviated form of the whole body treatment for more than 40 different, frequently occurring health disharmonies are described in his book "Reiki for First Aid", Lotus Light · Shangri-La, Twin Lakes, WI 1995.

29) In the higher degrees of Rainbow Reiki, there is an entire range of possibilities for working with advanced Reiki techniques in a very time-saving and specific manner. These can frequently—but definitely not always—replace the whole body treatment.

30) From: "Reiki Fire" by Frank Arjava Petter, Lotus Light · Shangri-La, Twin Lakes, WI, 1998, third edition.

31) See "Tao of Money" by Walter Lübeck, Lotus Press · Shangri-La, Twin Lakes, WI, 2000.

32) Stuhlmacher, J.: "Das große Handbuch der Naturheilkunde", Windpferd Verlag, Aitrang, Germany, 1998.

Hawayo Takata's Reiki Certificate

CERTIFICATE

THIS IS TO CERTIFY that Mrs. Hawayo Takata, an American citizen born in the Territory of Hawaii, after a course of study and training in the Usui system of Reiki healing undertaken under my personal supervision during a visit to Japan in 1935 and subsequently, has passed all the tests and proved worthy and capable of administering the treatment and of conferring the power of Reiki on others.

THEREFORE I, Dr. Chujiro Hayashi, by virtue of my authority as a Master of the Usui Reiki system of drugless healing, do hereby confer upon Mrs. Hawayo Takata the full power and authority to practice the Reiki system and to impart to others the secret knowledge and the gift of healing under this system.

MRS. HAWAYO TAKATA is hereby certified by me as a practitioner and Master of Dr. Usui's Reiki system of healing, at this time the only person in the United States authorized to confer similar powers on others and one of the thirteen fully qualified as a Master of the profession.

Signed by me this 21st day of February, 1938, in the city and county of Honolulu, territory of Hawaii.

(SIGNED) Chujiro Hayashi

Witness to his signature:
Yoshio Hanao

TERRITORY OF HAWAII, }
City and County of Honolulu. } ss.

On this 21st day of February A. D. 1938 before me personally appeared
. . . . (DR.) CHUJIRO HAYASHI . . . .
to me known to be the person described in and who executed the foregoing instrument and acknowledged that HE executed the same as HIS free act and deed.

W. Silva
Notary Public, First Judicial Circuit,
Territory of Hawaii.

Hawayo Takata's Lecture Ad

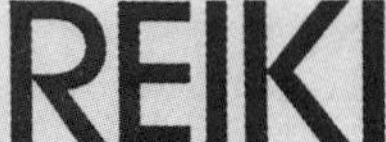

Reiki (ray-kee) means Universal Life Energy and is the endless source of healing power. Initiation through the master's meditation will attune you to the source of healing power ... for self-healing and for the healing of others.

CLASSES BY MRS. HAWAYO TAKATA -- THE ONLY TEACHER OF THE USUI SYSTEM OF REIKI HEALING IN THE WORLD TODAY

MRS. HAWAYO TAKATA of Honolulu, Hawaii, will conduct classes in Reiki healing -- the art of healing through "cosmic energy" -- in the Chicago suburban area:

May 30 - June 3, 1976 at the home of Mrs. Virginia Samdahl, 419 Winnemac, Park Forest, IL., 312/748-6639. Please phone for details.

SAC sponsored classes (see registration form below) are as follows:

June 6 - 10, 1976: Classes in Lockport, Illinois (southwest)

INTRODUCTORY LECTURE Open to Public: Sunday, June 6th at 7:30 P.M. at the Lemont United Methodist Church, 25 Custer, Lemont, IL. Classes for students on Monday thru Thursday at 7:30 P.M. at home of Ethel Lombardi, 93 Spring Creek Rd., Rt. 5, Lockport, IL. PHONE: 815/838-8218.

June 13 - 17, 1976: Classes in Golf, IL (northwest near Glenview)

INTRODUCTORY LECTURE Open to Public: Sunday, June 13th at 7:30 P.M. at the St. John's Lutheran Church, 4707 W. Pratt, Lincolnwood (Touhy exit from Edens, 4 blks S to Pratt, 1 blk east). Classes for students on Monday thru Thursday at 7:30 P.M. at home of Paul & Marikay Johnson, 45 Overlook Dr, Golf, IL. (1 blk N of Golf Rd & Waukegan Rd to Overlook Dr.; east to Clyde). 312/729-0320.

The introductory lecture is for students and the general public. Regular class sessions leading to the first degree will be held on four consecutive evenings (day classes are possible if enough people enroll). The cost is $125 per person ($75 for a spouse). Please indicate your interest in the class session on the registration form below and mail with your deposit to SAC. Reiki healers interested in the second degree, please contact SAC and make your intentions known (729-9490).

- -

__ Yes, I am interested in joining a Reiki class and I enclose my $25.00 deposit. Please reserve a place for me

__ June 6 - 10, 1976 in Lockport (Ethel Lombardi's home)

__ June 13-17, 1976 in Golf, Ill. (Paul Johnson's home)

__ I would prefer an afternoon class if it becomes available.

Name ______________________ Address ______________________

City/State/Zip ______________________ Phone ______________________

Make Checks Payable to:

SPIRITUAL ADVISORY COUNCIL
1701 LAKE AVENUE, GLENVIEW, ILLINOIS 60025, 312/729-9490

Letter from the Doshisha University

December 17, 1991

Mr. William L. Rand
President
The Center for Spiritual Development
20782 Knobwoods Dr., Suite 203
Southfield, MI 48086 U.S.A.

Dear Mr. Rand:

First, you could get some informations on the history of Doshisha University from enclosed photocopies made from Doshisha University Catalogue and The Doshisha.
Second, I, aided by chief archivist, checked the mentioned person, Mikao Usui with the related documents in vain;List of graduate students on Doshisha Alumni Bulletin, Literatures relating to J.H.Neesima, and List of faculty and clerical members in those days. I just found out he was never the presidentof Doshisha. And the name never appeared, and neither left any traces on them.
So I am afraid I cannot provide you any information.

Sincerely,

Itsuro Nishida

Itsuro Nishida
Head, Public Services
Center for Academic Information
(formerly Library)
Doshisha University
Kyoto 602, Japan

Letter from the University of Chicago

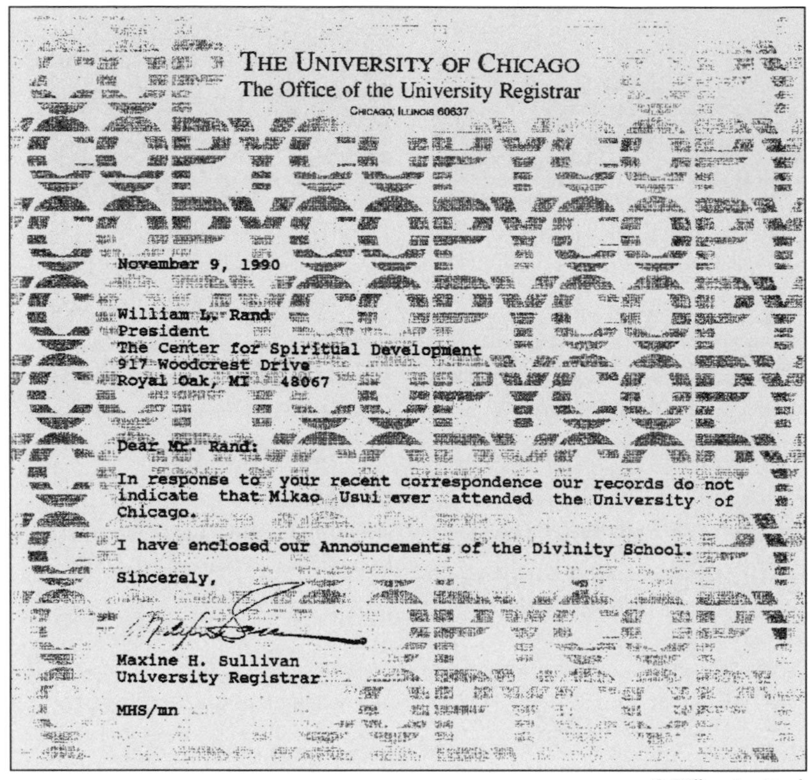

THE UNIVERSITY OF CHICAGO
The Office of the University Registrar
CHICAGO, ILLINOIS 60637

November 9, 1990

William L. Rand
President
The Center for Spiritual Development
917 Woodcrest Drive
Royal Oak, MI 48067

Dear Mr. Rand:

In response to your recent correspondence our records do not indicate that Mikao Usui ever attended the University of Chicago.

I have enclosed our Announcements of the Divinity School.

Sincerely,

Maxine H. Sullivan
University Registrar

MHS/mn

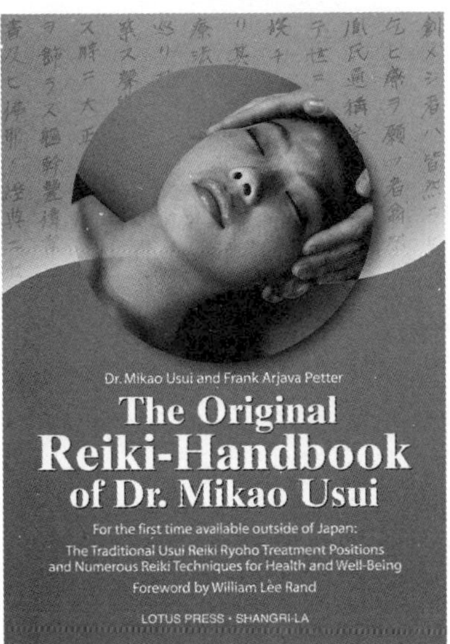

Dr. Mikao Usui and Frank A. Petter

The Original Reiki Handbook of Dr. Mikao Usui

The Traditional Usui Reiki Ryoho Treatment Positions and Numerous Reiki Techniques for Health and Well-Being

For the first time available outside of Japan: This book will show you the original hand positions from Dr. Usui's handbook. It has been illustrated with 100 colored photos to make it easier to understand. The hand positions for a great variety of health complaints have been listed in detail, making it a valuable reference work for anyone who practices Reiki. Now, that the original handbook has been translated into English, Dr. Usui's hand positions and healing techniques can be studied directly for the first time. Whether you are an initiate or a master, if you practice Reiki you can expand your knowledge dramatically as you follow in the footsteps of a great healer.

80 pages · 100 photos · $14.95
ISBN 0-914955-57-8

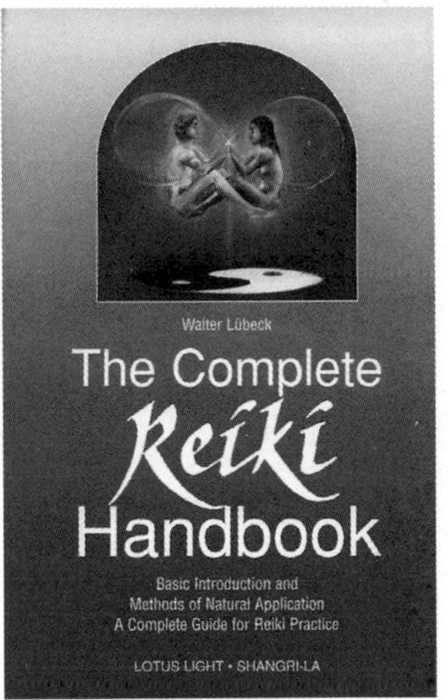

Walter Lübeck

The Complete Reiki Handbook

Basic Introduction and Methods of Natural Application—A Complete Guide for Reiki Practice

This handbook is a complete guide for Reiki practice and a wonderful tool for the necessary adjustment to the changes inherent in a new age. The author's style of natural simplicity, much appreciated by the readers of his many bestselling books, wonderfully complements this basic method for accessing universal life energy. He shares with us, as only a Reiki master can, the personal experience accumulated in his years of practice. Lovely illustrations of the different positions make the information as easily accessible visually as the author's direct and undogmatic style of writing. This work also offers a synthesis of Reiki and many other popular forms of healing.

192 pages · $14.95
ISBN 0-941524-87-6

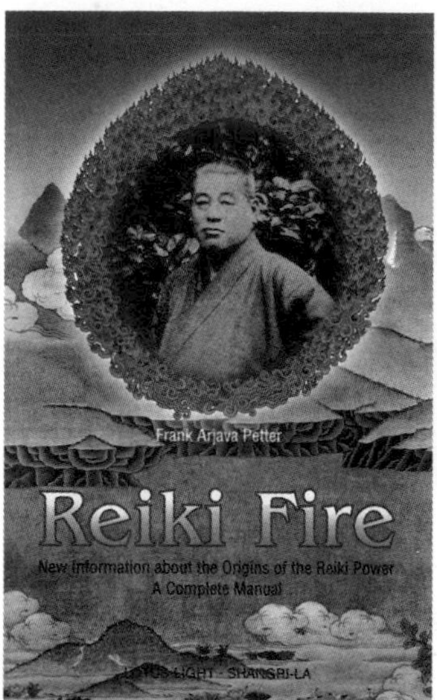

Frank Arjava Petter

Reiki Fire

New Information about the Origins of the Reiki Power—A Complete Manual

The origin of Reiki has come to be surrounded by many stories and myths. The author, an independent Reiki Master practicing in Japan, immerses it in a new light as he traces Usui-san's path back through time with openness and devotion. He meets Usui's descendants and climbs the holy mountain of his enlightenment. Reiki, shaped by Shintoism, is a Buddhist expression of Qigong, whereby Qigong depicts the teaching of life energy in its original sense. An excellent textbook, fresh and rousing in its spiritual perspective, this is an absolutely practical Reiki guide. The heart, the body, the mind, and the esoteric background, are all covered here.

128 pages · $12.95
ISBN 0-914955-50-0

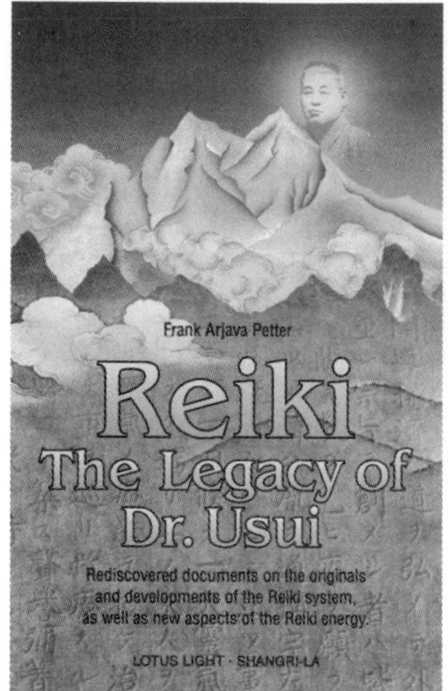

Frank Arjava Petter

Reiki—The Legacy of Dr. Usui

Rediscovered Documents on the Origins and Developments of the Reiki System, as well as New Aspects of the Reiki Energy

A great deal has been written and said to date about the history of Reiki and his founder. Now Frank Ajarva Petter, a Reiki Master who lives in Japan, has come across documents that quote Mikao Usui's original words. Questions that his students asked and he answered throw light upon Usui's very personal view of the teachings. Materials meant as the basis for his student's studies round off the entire work. A family tree of the Reiki successors is also included here. In a number of essays, Frank Ajarva Petter also discusses topics related to Reiki and the viewpoints of an independent Reiki teacher.

128 pages · $12.95
ISBN 0-914955-56-X

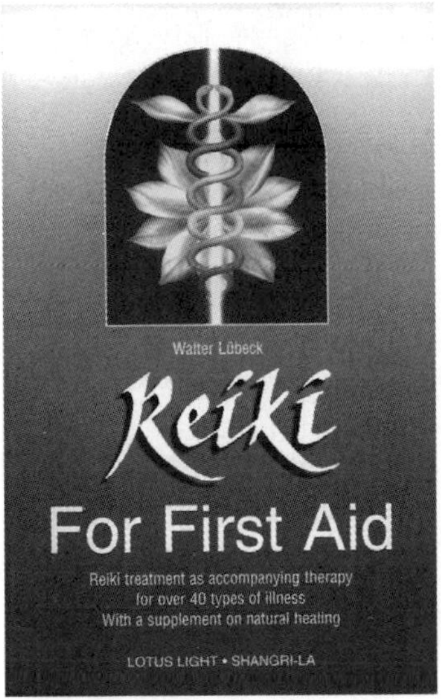

Walter Lübeck

Reiki For First Aid

Reiki Treatment as Accompanying Therapy for over 40 Types of Illness With a Supplement on Natural Healing

Reiki For First Aid offers much practical advice for applying the universal life force in everyday health care. The book includes Reiki treatments for over forty types of illness, supplemented with natural-healing applications and a detailed description of the relationship between Reiki and nutrition.

Reiki Master Walter Lübeck gives extensive instructions on topics ranging from Reiki whole-body treatments to special positions. These special Reiki treatment positions are an important contribution to the field of natural healing.

160 pages · $14.95

ISBN 0-914955-26-8

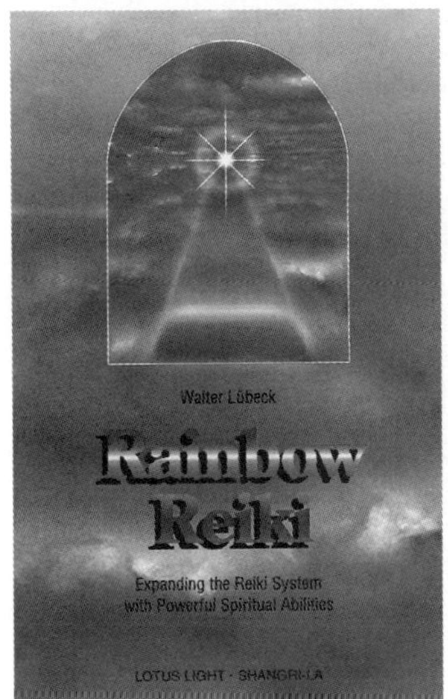

Walter Lübeck

Rainbow Reiki

Expanding the Reiki System with Powerful Spiritual Abilities

Rainbow Reiki gives us a wealth of possibilities to achieve completely new and different things with Reiki than taught in the traditional system. Walter Lübeck has tested these new methods in practical application for years and teaches them in his courses.

Making Reiki Essences, performing guided aura and chakra work, connecting with existing power places and creating new personal ones, as well as developing Reiki Mandalas, are all a part of this system. This work is accompanied by plants devas, crystal teachers, angels of healing stones, and other beings of the spiritual world.

184 pages · $14.95

ISBN 0-914955-28-4

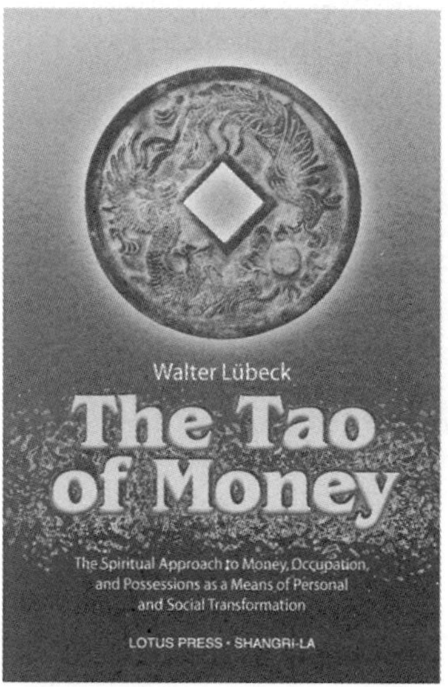

Walter Lübeck

The Tao of Money

The Spiritual Approach to Money, Occupation, and Possessions as a Means of Personal and Social Transformation

The Tao of Money explores how to heal material consciousness. For author Walter Lübeck, money can be equated with energy, something that manifests itself in every conceivable manner. This fascinating book about money contains many exercises on its spiritual meaning, work, occupation, and much more. How you treat money in your everyday life also expresses the inner state of your soul.

To a large extent, money has a deep spiritual dimension: Money activates the root chakra, wealth sets the love-of-life chakra into motion, and work affects the power chakra and the heart chakra. You can awaken the expression chakra through your job and use possessions to increase your kundalini energy. Discover what type of money person you are.

160 pages · $14.95
ISBN 0-914955-62-4

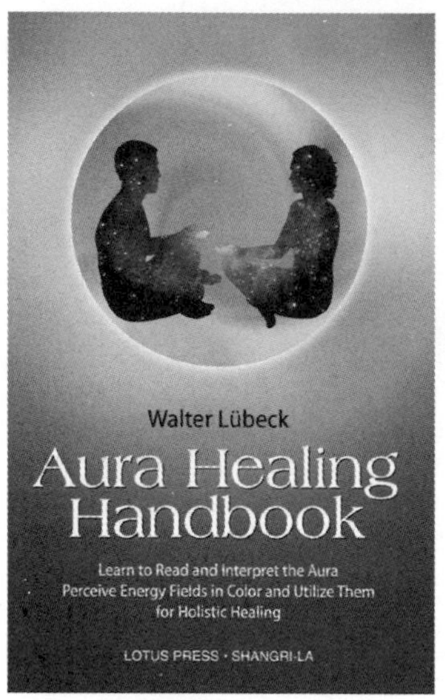

Walter Lübeck

Aura Healing Handbook

Learn to Read and Interpret the Aura · Perceive Energy Fields in Color and Utilize Them for Holistic Healing

Anyone can basically learn to see auras. Walter Lübeck's Aura Healing Handbook is a step-by-step instruction manual: By increasing your sensitivity for subtle vibrations, it will ultimately lead you into the fascinating world of seeing auras.

The author explains how to develop your "psychic" powers. He describes the different ways in which you can use these powers and the areas to which you can appl y them. As a result, you can see subtle energies and they will reveal their secrets to you.

Aura reading serves as a diagnostic aid in recognizing health disorders long before they manifest themselves within the body in the form of pain or unwellness. Reading the aura is the first step to healing your energies and emotions in the subtle realm.

224 pages · $15.95
ISBN 0-914955-61-6

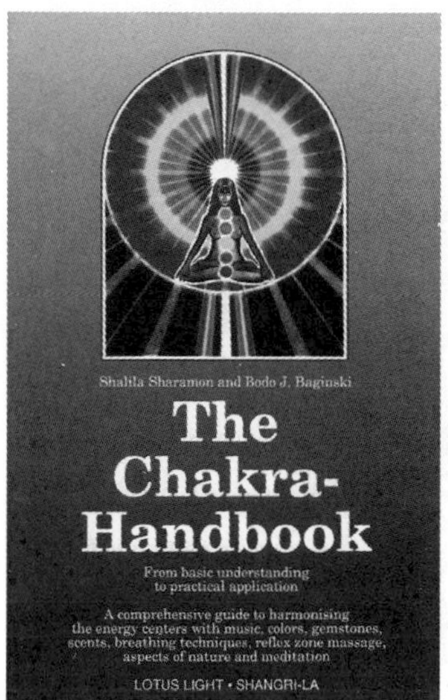

Shalila Sharamon and
Bodo J. Baginski

The Chakra Handbook

From Basic Understanding to Practical Application

Knowledge of the energy centers provides us with deep, comprehensive insight into the effects the subtle powers have on the human organism. This book vividly describes the functioning of the energy centers. For practical work with the chakras this book offers a wealth of possibilities: the use of sounds, colors, gemstones, and fragrances with their own specific effects, augmented by meditation, breathing techniques, foot reflexology massage of the chakra points, and the instilling of universal life energy. The description of nature experiences, yoga practices, and the relationship of each indiviual chakra to the zodiac additionally provides inspiring and valuable insight.

192 pages · $14.95
ISBN 0-941524-85-X

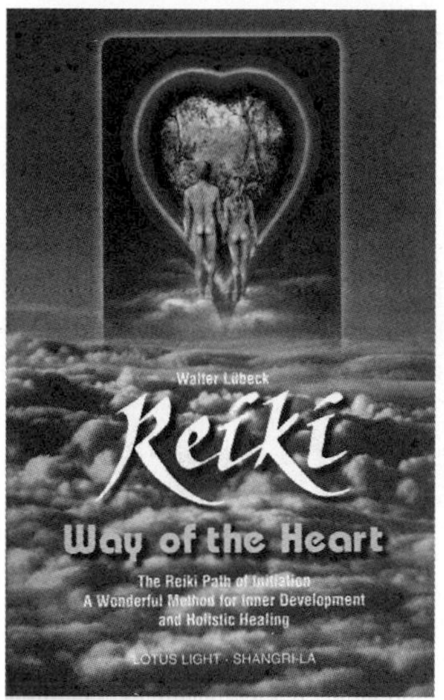

Walter Lübeck

Reiki—Way of the Heart

The Reiki Path of Initiation
A Wonderful Method for Inner Development and Holistic Healing

Reiki—Way of the Heart is for everyone interested in the opportunities and experiences offered by this very popular esoteric path of perception, based on easily learned exercises conveyed by a Reiki Master to students in three degrees.
If you practice Reiki, the use of universal life energy to heal oneself and others, you will have the possibility of receiving direct knowledge about your personal development, health, and transformation. Walter Lübeck also presents a good survey of various Reiki schools and shows how Reiki can be applied successfully in many areas of life.

192 pages · $14.95
ISBN 0-941524-91-4

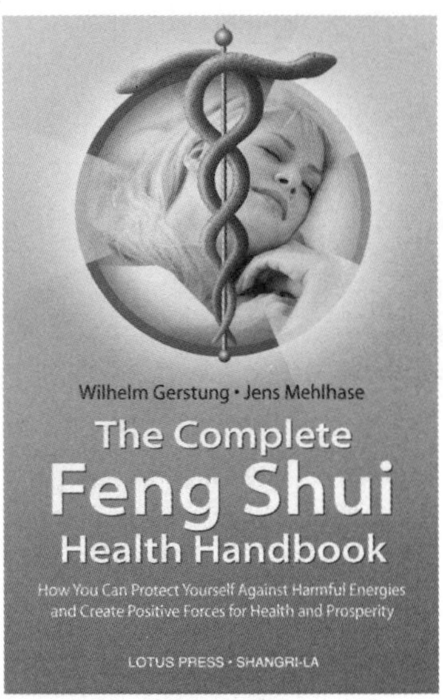

Wilhelm Gerstung and Jens Mehlhase

The Complete Feng Shui Health Handbook

How You Can Protect Yourself Against Harmful Energies and Create Positive Forces for Health and Prosperity

The authors are experienced Feng Shui practitioners and consultants. They explain how the invisible energies of Feng Shui can be directly measured and evaluated using a tensor (single-handed dowser) or pendulum. This means that you can use Feng Shui to understand many health problems by relating them to energy imbalances.

This fascinating handbook provides a wealth of graphics and practical information, which help design every home in such a way that it becomes a source of energy, allowing everybody to relax and re-energize himself. The authors integrate their many years of research and extensive knowledge of energies in the home, and particularly the sleeping area, with the Western science of underground watercourses and grids.

248 pages · $16.95

ISBN 0-914955-60-8

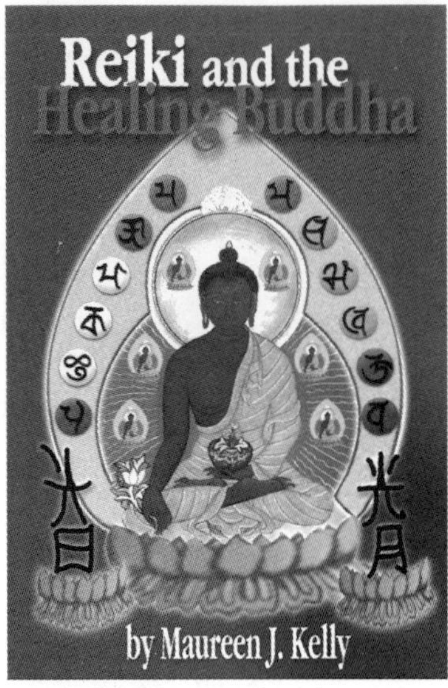

Maureen Kelly

Reiki and the Healing Buddha

The origins of Reiki go back to the Buddhist tradition in the distant past. One of the forms of Buddha revered in Tibet and China was the "Healing Buddha". Esoteric meanings are associated with the Reiki symbols and principles. These meanings originate in the Buddhist concepts of healing. While Dr. Usui rediscovered Reiki by studying Buddhist sutras, much of the hidden, esoteric sense has been overlooked in the subsequent teaching of Reiki to Christian practitioners in the West. The underlying symbology and esoteric sense provide new deeper understanding to the action and principles of Reiki and can enhance the practice, regardless of your own particular religious or philosophical background. This book reconnects Reiki with its Buddhist antecedents and provides both the experienced practitioner and the interested lay person with new insights and viewpoints on Reiki.

216 pages · $15.95

ISBN 0-914955-92-6

Reiki
The Healing Relaxation

*M*usic recommended by leading Reiki masters

Gently flowing sounds, all tuned in the spirit and rhythm of Reiki. While listening to *Reiki* and *Reiki—Light Touch*, bells will tell you when to change the treatment positions. *The Heart of Reiki* is composed in a completely intuitive timing and the *Chakra Meditation* supports the flow of infinite energy. *Elements of Rejuvenation* is mostly suited for effective qi exercises.

MERLIN'S MAGIC
Elements of Rejuvenation
Qi Gong Energy of Healing
CD 41094 · ISBN 0-910261-43-1 · $17.95

MERLIN'S MAGIC
Reiki
CD 41025 · ISBN 0-910261-87-3 · $17.95
CASS 42025 · ISBN 0-910261-81-4 · $10.95

MERLIN'S MAGIC ·
SHALILA SHARAMON / BODO J. BAGINSKI
Chakra Meditation (audio)
CD 41004 · ISBN 0-910261-57-1 · $17.95
CASS 42004 · ISBN 0-910261-80-6 · $10.95

MERLIN'S MAGIC
Reiki – Light Touch
CD 41055 · ISBN 0-910261-85-7 · $17.95
CASS 42055 · ISBN 0-910261-79-2 · $10.95

MERLIN'S MAGIC
The Heart of Reiki
CD 41081 · ISBN 0-910261-52-0 · $17.95
CASS 42081 · ISBN 0-910261-53-9 · $10.95

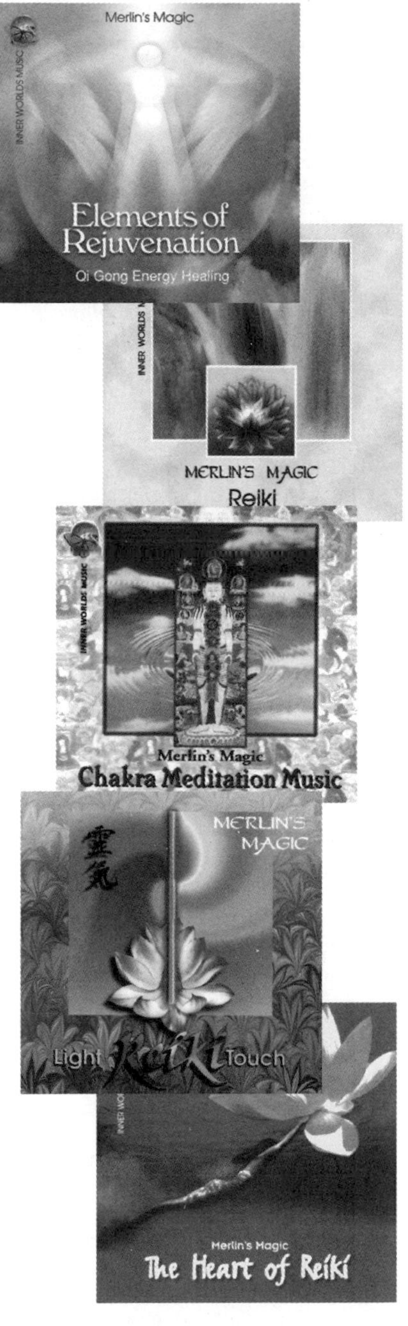

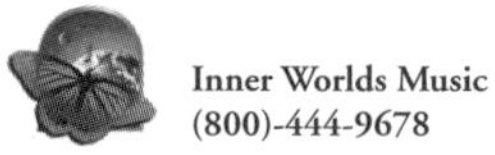

Inner Worlds Music
(800)-444-9678

Herbs and other natural health products and information are often available at natural food stores or metaphysical bookstores. If you cannot find what you need locally, you can contact one of the following sources of supply.

Sources of Supply:

The following companies have an extensive selection of useful products and a long track-record of fulfillment. They have natural body care, aromatherapy, flower essences, crystals and tumbled stones, homeopathy, herbal products, vitamins and supplements, videos, books, audio tapes, candles, incense and bulk herbs, teas, massage tools and products and numerous alternative health items across a wide range of categories.

WHOLESALE:

Wholesale suppliers sell to stores and practitioners, not to individual consumers buying for their own personal use. Individual consumers should contact the RETAIL supplier listed below. Wholesale accounts should contact with business name, resale number or practitioner license in order to obtain a wholesale catalog and set up an account.

Lotus Light Enterprises, Inc.

P. O. Box 1008
Silver Lake, WI 531 70 USA
262 889 8501 (phone)
262 889 8591 (fax)
800 548 3824 (toll free order line)

RETAIL:

Retail suppliers provide products by mail order direct to consumers for their personal use. Stores or practitioners should contact the wholesale supplier listed above.

Internatural

33719 116th Street
Twin Lakes, WI 53181 USA
800 643 4221 (toll free order line)
262 889 8581 office phone
WEB SITE: www.internatural.com

Web site includes an extensive annotated catalog of more than 10,000 products that can be ordered "on line" for your convenience 24 hours a day, 7 days a week.